- HOW CAN I TELL IF A KITTEN IS HEALTHY?

- WHAT TOYS ARE SAFE FOR MY CAT TO PLAY WITH?

- WHAT—AND HOW MUCH—SHOULD I FEED MY CAT?

- WHAT CAN I DO ABOUT SHEDDING?

The answers to these questions—and many more—are now available from cat expert Mordecai Siegal . . . in this handy guide for the new cat owner. Find out what you need to know to keep your cat purring happily . . . he'll love you for it!

HAPPY KITTENS, HAPPY CATS

HAPPY KITTENS, HAPPY CATS

MORDECAI SIEGAL

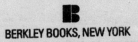

BERKLEY BOOKS, NEW YORK

HAPPY KITTENS, HAPPY CATS

A Berkley Book / published by arrangement with the author

PRINTING HISTORY
Berkley edition / March 1993

ISBN: 0-425-13765-1

A BERKLEY BOOK ® TM 757,375
Berkley Books are published by The Berkley Publishing Group, 200 Madison Avenue, New York, New York 10016.
The name "BERKLEY" and the "B" logo
are trademarks belonging to Berkley Publishing Corporation.

PRINTED IN THE UNITED STATES OF AMERICA

10   9   8   7   6

With awesome love for my son Jasper,
who loves cats even more than baseball.

ACKNOWLEDGMENTS

The author would like to express his deep gratitude to the staff and management of the Cat Fanciers' Association, Inc., for immeasurable help and encouragement with the CFA breed standards. In particular, many thanks to Thomas H. Dent, Executive Director; Michael W. Brim, Director of Public Relations; Connie Sellitto, Programmer/Analyst; Allene Sergi, Associate Director; and to Rosemary Suss, Senior Administrator.

Many thanks also goes to Kathy Lord for her invaluable grooming information. Much appreciation (and respect) goes to Carol Rothfeld, President of the Empire Cat Club and to Donna Davis, CFA All-Breed Judge for their invaluable advice and help.

CONTENTS

HAPPY KITTENS, HAPPY CATS

PART ONE

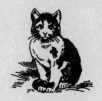

Caring for Your Cat

CHAPTER ONE

Getting a Cat

Most people think of cats as furry humans with tails. They are wrong. Although taking care of a cat is easy and uncomplicated, there is much you should learn if you want to find the right one and raise it properly. A cat can be the most unchanging member of your family, who will never grow up, leave home, and forget to call or write. For some, cats are the children they never had (or wanted), and because of this, they may fail to recognize the differences between cats and people. When you are entrusted with the responsibility of a cat, you should learn about its unique needs as a remarkable animal. By learning how to take *proper* care of your cat you can improve the quality of its life, which in turn will improve the quality of yours.

The new cat owner needs information. For example, a cat has totally different nutritional requirements from other animals; food meant for humans or dogs can be harmful to the health of the domestic feline. A cat's life may hang in the balance if an inexperienced owner does not know how to prevent illnesses that are life-threatening or how to recognize danger signs. And there is a lot to be learned about grooming and bathing, fleas, allergies, obesity, first aid. And what about training, housebreaking, kittenhood, and feline behavior? It may come as a surprise to learn that few cats are as independent and enterprising as Garfield, and most need more help than you can imagine. If cats could speak, they would tell us what they really need, and that just might surprise all of us.

What puzzles most people about cats is the contradiction between their independent behavior and their need for human care. All cats succumb to the whir of the can opener and the thrill of a well-stroked back. They want to be fed every day at the same time, groomed, played with, and given lots of affection and attention. These facts clash with the accepted image of cats.

The contradiction between their independent bearing and their needful demands can be attributed to their lives in the human environment. It has now been thousands of generations since domestic cats left their initial existence in the wild and willingly stepped into the relative safety and comfort of the human home. As domestic animals they have been bred selectively for specific looks and traits considered desirable by humans, and they have been encouraged to respond to the kindness and indulgence of their human "parents." The pussycats we live with are very different from their wild relatives, who must fend for themselves and live off the land. Our cats are eternal teenagers, suspended somewhere between childhood and maturity. They are indeed independent, but only to a point.

WHERE TO GET A CAT

Cats are everywhere; it's easy to get one. For better or for worse, there is never a shortage of kittens, and many of them are free. Taking a kitten off your neighbor's hands may seem like a good idea at the time, but it is not the only way to get a cat, and it isn't necessarily the best way. It all depends on what kind of cat you want, how much you are willing to spend, and whether you want to show the cat or just have it share its unique life with you. For most of us, a new cat's destiny is to become a member of the family, and that's a big deal. Anything that important should certainly involve a little of your time and good judgment. Acquiring a cat is an important step.

The source of your cat and how you select it have a great influence on the length and quality of its life. You may pay more money for a healthy, beautiful cat of your choice, but it may cost you far less in the long run in veterinary bills. Acquiring a healthy cat of sound temperament and emotional stability does not depend on luck alone. The beauty of a cat is also a consideration. There are more than forty recognized breeds to choose from in addition to the many variations among random-bred cats. See Part Two, *The Show Standards of the Cat Fanciers' Association*, to learn more about cat breeds.

Personal taste and compatibility are an important part of selecting a cat. Bear in mind that you will be living with your new family member between one and two decades. It is not a good idea to simply accept the first kitten you see. When looking at the kitten in front of you, try to imagine what it will be like as a grown cat.

If you are like most people looking for a cat, you simply want one that you are going to enjoy as a companion. However, you may want one that will compete successfully in cat shows, or one that will be part of a planned breeding program. Without question, however, more cats are purchased as pets than for any other reason. No matter what your desire, you will still want the best cat possible, and it helps to know where you can find it.

There are many ways to acquire a cat. If you wish to adopt one, you can visit an animal shelter or seek those who rescue cats as a major activity in their lives. (They're out there!) You can also go to one of the thousands of private catteries that have breeding programs focusing on one or two pure breeds. Ever since the popularity of cats began to soar, more and more pet shops have begun selling kittens on a regular basis. Bear in mind that catteries, pet shops, shelters, and adoption sources are only as good as the people running them *and* where *they* got their cats. Ask questions and pursue thorough answers. You'll see that your choices will range from excellent to horrible. The following sections will help you with this evaluation.

Adoption Agencies

The traditional method of adopting a cat is to go to an established animal welfare agency that is owned or supported by local government. Many of these groups are known as the SPCA, or the Society for the Prevention of Cruelty to Animals. These should not be confused with the *ASPCA,* which is a New York City–based organization with local animal welfare functions and some national educational and promotional activities.

There are also animal rescue and adoption agencies that are private, nonprofit organizations, institutional in nature and with impressive reputations. There are hundreds of such significant organizations throughout North America, such as the Tree House Animal Foundation in Chicago; the Hawaiian Humane Society; the Humane Society of New York; Pet Pride in Pacific Palisades, California; St. Hubert's Giralda in Chatham Township, New Jersey; and others, too numerous to mention.

Considered the best bargain available, purchasing a cat from an adoption agency, whether it is city-owned or not, varies in cost from community to community. Still, the price is always reasonable and the animals are usually in good health. If a kitten is too young for neutering when you get it, the organization often requires that you agree to have the surgical procedure done at the proper time. Many of the organizations will have performed the procedure before the cat is ready to leave the shelter.

Aside from economics, another important reason for getting your cat from such an agency is to rescue it from possibly being put to sleep. A shelter is the most worthwhile animal source one can use. It affords cat lovers a wide range of choice plus the opportunity to provide safety and comfort for a homeless animal. There are simply not enough homes for the surplus of cats and dogs that become lost and abandoned or are born unwanted. Homeless animals fortunate enough to make it to a shelter spend the remainder of their lives waiting to be adopted or euthanized.

Most of the wonderful cats and kittens at adoption agencies have no pedigree and are of unknown heritage. Still, they are as beautiful and delightful as any feline anywhere. Of course, now and again, there does appear a pure-breed cat. So, whether you're looking for a kitten or an adult, alley cat or aristocrat, check with all the agencies in your community before spending a lot of money. Most adoption agencies are listed in the Yellow Pages under *Animal Shelters*.

Among the hundreds of animal welfare agencies there are the major organizations that can offer a wide range of services including medical care. These are sufficiently staffed with veterinarians, trained veterinary assistants, administrators, animal handlers, peace officers, informational hotline staff, and so on. There are also many smaller operations that are exclusively staffed with volunteers who are caring workers. Many of them are unfunded, unchartered, and in some cases, unlicensed. Although it is impossible to asses the quality of their efforts in general terms, it can be said that their work is often effective.

Another source of adoption is the loosely formed network of private individuals who rescue abandoned and lost cats and dogs. They often advertise in local newspapers or by word of mouth and offer pets free of charge to those who are willing to give them good homes. They seldom allow an unspayed or unneutered cat to leave their protection and spend great amounts of their own money for the surgical procedures. These well-intentioned volunteers are sometimes thought of as eccentric and given such epithets as ''cat ladies'' or ''cat crazies.'' Whether or not one approves of the extent of their involvement with rescue efforts or their sense of priorities, the fact remains that these people rescue otherwise doomed animals by the thousands. They often give the cats medical attention, have them altered, fed, and cleaned and placed in good homes. You can find such volunteers in your community. The animal you receive will have gotten a clean bill of health from a veterinarian, and the chore and expense of altering will have been taken care of. There is usually very little or no money involved, although a contribution is appreciated.

Many who have adopted cats from these various sources have described the experience as pleasant, exciting, interesting, and heartwarming. The purrs and meows of a cat being taken to its new home can be interpreted as the sound of gratitude.

The Veterinarian's Office

Believe it or not, veterinarians are indirectly (and sometimes directly) responsible for placing many cats and kittens in new homes. In countless veterinary clinics, hospitals, and private practices, there is a bulletin board littered with dozens of notices about homeless kittens and cats. Vets have traditionally served their communities and their clientele as a catalyst for those who must find new homes for their pets and those who are looking for pets. They are another great source to consider when acquiring a new pet.

Breeders

The term breeder here does not include the "backyard breeder" who is most often someone who knows nothing about genetics or the concepts of selective and healthy breeding. They rarely know what they are doing. They are either trying to get rid of unwanted kittens or trying to make a few easy dollars. They are a detriment to the cause of animal population control and social responsibility. The barest health essentials are usually ignored, and it's anyone's guess as to the soundness of the resulting kittens. Acquiring a kitten from such a source is risky and only encourages such activities which add to the tragic problem of the over-population of pet animals.

Commercial breeders supply pet shops and specialty stores with kittens in both large and small quantities, depending on their operations. Some cater to the general public through advertising in newspapers. Commercial breeders may operate out of a farm, a garage, a basement, or even a large apartment. Profit is the only consideration, which brings into serious question the true quality and health of the animals being made available. It is only fair to state, however, that some commercial breeders are skilled, knowledgeable, and responsible, and function fairly and competently, while others are unprincipled and inhumane in their practices. If you visit such an operation, look for a clean setting. Are the cats and kittens healthy-looking? Are they in a sanitary, spacious confinement? Does anyone handle them gently and lovingly or pay the slightest attention to their needs? Do they appear to be well fed and given medical attention? Is there a record of immunization? Will the owner give you a written guarantee pertaining to the kitten's health?

Noncommercial breeders are usually members of the Cat Fancy, which means they have a cattery registered with a national cat association, breed pure-breed cats exclusively, register their kittens with the same national cat association, and compete in cat shows that are sanctioned by the cat association of choice. Such breeders are more than willing to show you the pedigree (printed family tree) of any kitten they have produced, along with the animal's registration papers.

They are more knowledgeable and ethical as a group than most other types of cat breeders. When you purchase a kitten from such a breeder, ask if the kittens are registered with any of the six major cat associations: the American Cat Association, the American Cat Fanciers' Association, the Canadian Cat Association, the Cat Fanciers' Association, the Cat Fanciers' Federation, or the International Cat Association.

Be prepared to spend more money for a kitten at one of these establishments than at any other. Although covering costs is an important consideration for noncommercial breeders, pride in the quality of their cats and the pleasure derived from them are among the major motivations of their activities. The reason kittens from a cattery cost more is the time and expense required to create beautiful cats that meet the breed standards set by the various national cat associations. (See Part Two, *The Show Standards of the Cat Fanciers' Association*.) Also, creating kittens that meet any high standard of health, temperament, and beauty is costly.

A common complaint from those who buy cats from commercial breeders is that the kittens often do not grow up looking like true representations of their breed. This is rarely a problem with kittens from noncommercial breeders because of the breeders' slavish devotion to the breed standard. This is the happy result of the practice of selective breeding based on

genetic principles. At a cattery pedigreed cats of the most
interesting and beautiful breeds are brought into the world with
the greatest selection and care possible. Catteries are an
important source when looking for a high-quality, pure-breed
kitten, though it is important to understand that some catteries
are better than others, and some are not at all satisfactory.

Catteries that are registered with a national cat association
are devoted to housing and mating pure-breed cats and producing pure-breed kittens. Most of them are established inside
the breeders' homes. Some breeders use a portion of their
living space to house their cats, while others have set up in a
garage or basement. Some catteries have elaborate buildings
that are separated from the breeders' homes and are used
exclusively for their cats. But if the cattery is clean, spacious,
and well ventilated, the size and luxury of its appearance is of
no significant importance. All that matters is the quality of its
animals and the reputation of its owners.

At a cattery litters of kittens are produced on a limited basis.
Individual kittens within the litter are sometimes categorized as
show quality, breeding quality, or *pet quality.* A *pet quality*
kitten is the least expensive one you can buy at a cattery.
Although it closely resembles its breed, it may have one or
more "faults" that would make it noncompetitive in the show
ring. Only a breeder or show judge may notice these imper-
fections, such as the wrong length of coat or ears that are
slightly too small or slightly too large, and so on. In every other
way, the kitten may be wonderful, in looks and temperament.
A kitten that is referred to as *breeding quality* comes very close
to the standard for its breed. For complicated reasons beyond
the scope of this book such a kitten may not be qualified to
compete for championship status in the show ring, but these
kittens are fine for serious breeding programs. Occasionally
they are purchased as pets. *Show quality* kittens are those that
appear to compare well to the written standard of their breed.
They have the best chance to become a Champion, Grand
Champion, or even win a national award. These are the most

expensive cats at a cattery and will sell for hundreds and, in some instances, thousands of dollars.

A proper cattery must have a separate area for newborn kittens, an isolation area for sick cats or newcomers, an area with cages for females, and another one for males (to prevent indiscriminate mating). The cages should be of adequate size to provide room for movement and comfort. A sensible breeder allows the cats to play outside the cages for specific periods during the day, although the males never mix with the females.

The serious cattery operator maintains strict standards of hygiene by keeping clean cages and litter pans and adequate ventilation, light, and odor control. All cats and kittens must be immunized and receive medical attention when necessary. The experienced cattery operator understands that distance between cats reduces the opportunity for infections and exposure to harmful bacteria and viruses; physical barriers such as cages, fences, and walls prevent cats from actual contact. Proper ventilation is necessary to prevent the spread of disease. A humid room containing many cats without a good air exchange promotes the transmission of communicable diseases. Fresh outside air is desirable. Circulating air from a ventilating system or air conditioner are necessary in a cattery.

Clean floors free of many infections require a daily mopping with a solution consisting of one part bleach to thirty-two parts water (1:32), followed by a rinsing with clear water. All walls, doors, windowsills, ceilings, light fixtures, and fans should be washed with the 1:32 bleach/water solution once a week. Although unneutered male cats spray their cages and walls with pungent-smelling urine, you should not be confronted with an unpleasant odor when entering a cattery. Proper sanitation and good ventilation remove most odors.

Most noncommercial cat breeders are also *exhibitors*, which means they enter their own cats for competition at cat shows. This is the primary reason for establishing and maintaining a cattery. The idea is to develop a line of pure-breed cats and then enter them in cat shows and see how well they do. The activity is part hobby, part sport.

A cattery need not win many First Place ribbons to produce outstanding cats. However, exhibitor-breeders who enter their cats in shows are exposed to the scrutiny of their peers. They lose all credibility if they are always identified with poor-quality cats. The merits of their cats reflect the merits of their breeding programs and of their catteries. A cat show is where a cattery establishes its reputation.

Pet Shops

Many pet shops sell pure-breed and mixed-breed kittens even though the proprietors understand the great availability from other sources. By charging lower prices for them, they hope to attract customers for the highly profitable cat supplies and paraphernalia. This includes cat food, toys, beds, cat furniture, scratch posts, over-the-counter remedies, and so on. Kittens are now seen in window displays as frequently as puppies, and pet shops are becoming a significant source of pure-breed kittens for prospective pet owners.

Some pet shops are operated by those who breed their own cats and maintain them until they are sold. Most shops, however, obtain their kittens from local commercial breeders or from various commercial sources of questionable origin and quality. Kittens in pet shops may be pure-breeds (with or without registration papers from a cat association) or mixed-breeds (which are unregisterable). A pure-breed kitten is eligible to be registered if both its parents were registered with a national cat association and registration papers exist to establish this. The hit-or-miss risk of getting a pet-shop kitten is much the same as that involved when getting a kitten from a backyard breeder. Good cats and bad cats have been purchased from pet shops. In all fairness, the same holds true for catteries and animal shelters.

If you go to a pet shop to buy a kitten, look the shop over carefully. The same standard for a noncommercial cattery should apply to a retail pet shop. The premises should be well lit, clean, cheerful, odor-free, and noticeably hygienic. There should be no more than two cats for each litter pan. The litter pans should be free of fecal matter, cleaned every day, and filled with fresh litter. The odor of cat urine should be slight.

Each cage or enclosure should house no more than one adult or two kittens and should provide ample room for the cat's comfort. Avoid purchasing kittens that have been placed together in large window displays. Lumping ten and twenty kittens together in the same enclosure is unhealthy and damaging to their personalities, affecting future behavior. One sick cat can make all the others sick as well. This is especially true about the spread of worms, fleas, lice, and mites. Observe how the shop employees handle the kittens. They must be gentle, affectionate, knowledgeable, and careful if the kittens are to grow into good-natured cats.

The problem with too many pet-shop purchases is that they are made on impulse rather than careful consideration and planning. That can be a disastrous mistake. It is less dangerous to buy a goldfish impulsively than a kitten. Salespeople at pet shops know how irresistible a kitten is once it's in your arms. Resist holding the kitten. Be prepared to say "No" if it does not answer your needs or desires.

SELECTING THE RIGHT CAT

Pure-breed or Mixed-breed?

When planning for a cat, your first decision is whether to get a pure-breed or mixed-breed. The differences between the two lie primarily in the fact that you can predict with reasonable certainty what a pure-breed kitten will look like as a grown cat. If you like the look and size of an adult Persian cat, you can be sure of getting that look when you buy a Persian kitten. The choice is a subjective one that must be based on personal preference and how much you can afford or want to spend.

Pure-breed cats have many features that fall within predictable boundaries: body size, body shape, length of the hair coat, coat color, coat pattern, shape of the head, tail type, and other factors. You can see what a pure-breed kitten will be like as an adult by examining a photograph of the breed. A mixed-breed cat, however, might grow up to be more or less than expected in size, shape, color, coat length, and all the rest.

Selecting a pure-breed cat also gives you the option to choose a breed that has predictable behavior traits you might prefer. Would you rather live with an outgoing cat that wants your attention or one that is aloof and requires solitude for the better part of the day? There are breeds that are very active and some that sleep much of the time. Which is better suited to your personality? Unless you are familiar with its parents, it is difficult to predict what a mixed-breed kitten's personality and temperament will be once it has grown into maturity. Of course, there are those who enjoy not knowing and prefer the surprise. For them this is the fun of getting a cat.

Male or Female?

The important differences between male and female cats are connected to sexual behavior. If you get a cat that has been surgically neutered or spayed, those differences become insignificant. Male or female cats that have been altered make ideal house pets. Both male and female cats that have *not* been surgically altered have appealing and unappealing behaviors associated with the differences between them. Which gender to decide on is a matter of personal choice.

Male cats are usually larger than females and a bit more aggressive and independent, with a tendency to be somewhat aloof. Unneutered (or *whole*) male cats must be mated on a frequent basis if they are to remain emotionally balanced. Because of their sexual needs, male cats will roam as far from home as necessary to pursue a female in heat. If not allowed out, males who can hear or smell a female in heat will pace back and forth vigorously, make a constant, loud, throaty growl, and make every effort to escape confinement. A male cat in this state may also spray sexually scented urine on walls, furniture, doors and other vertical objects. It is done to mark off territory and attract a female.

Whole male cats past puberty begin ''spraying'' around their territory (your home) with sexually scented urine that is unbearably pungent. They back up against walls, windows, and vertical objects when they are aroused or making territorial claims, lift their tails, and spray their scented urine. It is impossible to stop this behavior without surgical alteration and some behavior modification. A whole male cat will wander away from home whenever given the opportunity and will get into fights with other cats over territory and mating opportunities.

Female cats are usually more affectionate, stay home, and purr at the slightest touch. Unspayed females experience estrus (or "heat") at least twice a year, but many domestic female cats experience the estrus cycle on a continual basis or at least more than twice a year. This is probably the result of so many generations of domestication and its influences. The radical behavior changes of a female in estrus can be quite disturbing to the novice cat owner. Her postures and vocalizing are designed to attract the attention of nearby male cats. However, many humans exposed to this behavior may become frightened or disturbed by them. Sometimes sexual behaviors are confused with illness. During estrus the female cat secretes an odorous fluid intended to attract whole male cats for the purpose of mating. None of these behaviors remain once the female is surgically altered.

Whether to get a male or female cat will not be a difficult issue if you have your veterinarian spay the female cat (*ovariohysterectomy*) between six and eight months of age or sometime shortly after the first estrus cycle, or neuter the male cat (*castration*) between six and eight months of age. This will not only prevent undesirable sexual behavior but also unwanted pregnancies. These routine surgical procedures are inexpensive, humane, and necessary for a happy life with your new cat.

If you are not interested in the expense and bother of mating, pregnancy, birth, and kitten care, and it's best that you're not, then it doesn't matter whether you live with a male or female cat once you have your pet altered. Both genders are intelligent, beautiful, and pleasing in every way.

Select a Healthy Kitten

There is nothing more heartbreaking than learning to love a young cat only to lose it to poor health. The cost of veterinary care for a very sick cat can be quite high. For these reasons, it makes more sense to try to select a cat with the best chance for a long, healthy life. Your best opportunity for success lies in carefully observing the physical appearance and behavior of the kittens from which you must choose.

All kittens are adorable, and that makes it hard to pick one over the other. Chances are the one you like may not be the best one to choose. And do not be fooled by a pure-breed kitten's pedigree, either. Although a kitten's family tree is useful information, it has no ultimate bearing on its state of health. A medical record is far more useful.

You do not have to be a veterinarian to recognize the indications of good or bad health. You simply examine those elements of the feline body that can be seen. Although you have no way of knowing exactly what is going on inside the kitten's body, the outer appearances can tell you a great deal. You must look carefully at the kitten's coat, skin, eyes, nose, ears, teeth, stomach, anus, and genital areas.

The coat. The coat should be clean, have a slight sheen, and be free of fleas, lice, ticks, and mites. A dull or dirty coat means something is wrong. Bald or bare patches of skin showing through the coat may be indications of ringworm or mange. A healthy coat is full, lustrous, soft, and pleasant to the touch.

Skin. If you run your fingers through the coat, you will be able to see sections of the skin beneath and to feel what you cannot see. The skin should look and feel smooth with no apparent scaly areas or sores. A kitten's skin should also be free of tiny white or black particles; such particles indicate the presence of fleas. The white debris is flea eggs and the black debris is bits of coagulated blood and excrement left by the fleas.

Eyes. Be wary of liquid discharges from the eyes. Healthy eyes should be clear with no excessive watering, no white skin showing from the corners, no ulcers on the surface, which appear as small indentations, and no whitish scars from previous medical conditions. Look for any abnormalities, including soreness or swelling. A blue-eyed kitten with a white coat may be deaf.

Nose. A cool and slightly damp nose is best. There may be infection present if there is a liquid discharge from the nostrils. Sneezing, coughing, and runny nose could be signs of upper respiratory infections. Although a warm, dry nose is not necessarily an indication of poor health, it could indicate a poor environment for the kitten.

Ears. A kitten's ears must be free of discharges, dirt, and unpleasant odors. If a kitten constantly shakes its head and rubs its ears with its paws, look inside each one. If you see a dark, waxlike substance, it indicates the presence of ear mites, which are near-microscopic parasites that must be treated by a veterinarian. Mites create intense itching which can cause self-inflicted damage to the skin from the kitten's intense need to scratch the itching skin surface.

Teeth. A kitten's teeth should be clean and white. They are normal if they mesh properly with the upper incisors meeting the bottom incisors evenly. Incisors are the twelve small teeth in the front of the mouth, which are present by the fourth week. All twenty-six baby teeth should be present by the sixth week of age. (Adult cats have thirty teeth.) Pink gums indicate a healthy mouth. If the inside of the mouth or the gum tissue is pale or bluish in color, it could be a sign of anemia, which is a symptom itself of some other medical condition. A broken tooth could indicate that an accident took place recently. Loose teeth can be the sign of dental disease, vitamin deficiency, or "milk" teeth being exchanged for adult teeth. All adult teeth should be in place by six months of age.

Stomach. A swollen belly could indicate several medical conditions. However, a kitten with a distended stomach is most likely to be infected with internal parasites (worms), although it is sometimes caused by overeating. A bump on or near the navel of a kitten can be an umbilical hernia and requires medical attention.

Anus or external genital areas. These are the areas most likely to show the signs of internal parasites or a variety of medical conditions. The signs of roundworms are found in the kitten's feces. The presence of tapeworm infection is indicated by small, brownish segments in and around the anus and in the feces. Secretions, irritated tissue, and hair loss may indicate chronic diarrhea or serious viral infection.

The body. The stance of a healthy kitten should be straight and tall. Its legs must stand in a straight line from the trunk to the ground. A kitten's walk should be frisky, free and easy. Anything less in its movement could indicate a condition involving lameness.

Temperament. The best way to evaluate a kitten is to see it with its mother and its littermates. Observe how it interacts with the others; do not take one that is apparently shy, cowering away from you and the rest of the litter. A shy, nervous kitten is adorable and tugs at your heartstrings but can be a problem as an adult cat. Shy behavior usually leads to aggressive behavior later in life. A shy kitten is one that is frightened of people, other animals, noise, and change of every sort. Eventually, the fear creates aggressive behavior. Sometimes shy behavior is an indication of a medical problem or a poor state of health.

Avoid a kitten that is overaggressive, which is the other end of the behavior spectrum. A litter of kittens, especially past six weeks old, plays rough-and-tumble games like those of wild cubs. One kitten in the litter may be too tough for his own good and become the bully of the group. Such a kitten goes beyond the limits of exuberant play and displays hostile and potentially dangerous behavior. It is not difficult to distinguish play-fighting from the real thing. Watch for a sullen facial expression, stiffened body, straight legs and arched back, contracted pupils of the eyes, and ears flattened against the side of the head. A kitten in this state may be amusing because of its size but can be dangerous to the rest of the litter and eventually to humans as well. Watch how it deals with littermates and try to picture what this same behavior will be like when it is a full-grown cat. Pass on this kitten and choose another.

If a kitten catches your eye and appears to be a cat with normal temperament, watch it closely and try to relate to it. If your close presence does not frighten it, you're ahead of the game. Lift the kitten in your arms. If it doesn't struggle to get free, if it doesn't scratch or bite you, if it seems curious and friendly, this is probably the right cat to take home.

Choosing a cat should be a pleasant, enjoyable experience. Base your decision on the health, personality, and look of the kitten that has captured your attention. For a detailed description of the many cat breeds available, see Part Two, *The Official Show Standards of the Cat Fanciers' Association, Inc.*

CHAPTER TWO

A Kitten in Your Life

Cats get a bad press when it comes to love, dependency, and expressions of affection. Don't believe it. The typical house puss is a devoted tenderfoot when it comes to his own family. A domestic cat only seems to be independent and aloof. He is the great pretender. It is simply a matter of style. A cat is a needful creature and is no different than his colleague, the dog, in this respect. The similarity between cats and dogs lies in their exalted position as companions and friends.

There is nothing more demanding than a cat looking up at its human family, wanting to be held and petted. Yes, kittens and many adult cats crave loving affection in some physical form just as dogs do. When a kitten first arrives, everyone wants to get their hands on it and just love it to death. That is all well and good providing you hold down the enthusiasm a bit *and have properly prepared for the new arrival*. There are things that should be done *before* the kitten ever sets one paw inside the house. There are things to buy and things to do.

THINGS TO BUY

Litter Box, Cat Litter, and Rake

Litter boxes. When your new kitten or adult cat first enters your home, he is going to be disoriented and somewhat distressed. It is best to show him where he can relieve himself. By taking him directly to a litter box (and showing him what to do, if he is a kitten), you give him an opportunity to release his anxiety by scratching and eliminating. Please refer to Chapter Five, ''The Cat Train.'' The litter box is also the perfect place for a new cat to exercise his need to claim territory by marking it with the scent of his urine and feces. Urination and defecation mean more to an animal than the need to eliminate.

A litter box and the cat litter that goes in it are simply a toilet for your new pet. You have several options for this most essential bit of feline equipment. The most common cat box is a plastic cat pan ranging from eighteen inches to three feet in length. These come in many shapes and styles. Some are no more than a tray with high sides, and others come with a second piece that covers the pan. Those that have covers come with a snug opening for an entrance in the front. These afford the sense of privacy that many cats require, while also appealing to the human sense of aesthetics. Some litter boxes have air vents and filter systems at the top of the cover. Others offer a sifting tray that is helpful in removing solids. The variety and array of cat boxes is astounding (and very helpful to the new cat owner).

Cat litter. There is also a wide variety of cat litter that can go into the box. You can choose from products made of everything from plain granulated clay to chlorophyll-coated pellets. Cat litter products are made of materials that absorb urine, allow a cat to bury its feces, and may eliminate some of the odors. There are products that are heavily scented in order to disguise the strong odors coming from the box. Some products claim to be pH formulated, enabling them to *neutralize* the odors from cat urine rather than perfume them away. The newest brands of litter products offer a sandlike material that is super-absorbent and forms into clumps from liquid waste. The clumps are easily removed and enable the cat owner to rid the box of cat urine without actually changing the litter material. The cat owner need only replenish the litter that the clumps remove when they are discarded. Some experienced cat people simply use plain sand or gravel, while others may use shredded newspapers. These materials, however, must be changed several times a day. Your new cat will make the choice. Many cats refuse to use some types of litter and will relieve themselves on the floor until you find something they prefer. If you find something that the cat likes, stay with it.

The rake. You will need a rake-like tool to remove the solid waste material from the litter box every day. A very popular tool, basically a cooking utensil, has proved itself equally useful for the cat toilet. It is an aluminum (or plastic), spoonlike, slotted spatula about ten inches long. It will remove fecal material without taking the gravel and is inexpensive.

Bowls and Food

Bowls. The best water containers for cats are medium to small stainless steel bowls with shallow sides. They are easier to keep clean than plastic bowls and last forever. You can use the same kind of bowl for solid food. However, a flat dish for solid food is what a cat likes best. When you first offer food to your new cat, he is going to be cautious and somewhat doubtful about it. A flat dish will make it easier for him to examine and smell the food before eating it. A plate makes it easier for a small kitten to get to the food; it also allows a cat to do what it likes best with food—separate one morsel from the others. It is a good idea to place the food and water containers on a nonporous place mat to catch the spilt crumbs and water.

Plastic and ceramic bowls are also serviceable. However, some ceramic bowls are not fired at high enough temperatures in the kiln, thus allowing the lead content of the glaze to leach through and possibly cause lead poisoning. This is not usually a problem with American-made ceramics. Food and water should not be placed in the same container.

Food. Be prepared to feed your new cat soon after his arrival. The best idea is to obtain a one-week supply of the food that he has been getting. *Do not change your cat's diet suddenly.* A sudden change may cause diarrhea or vomiting at a time when your kitten needs maximum nutrition for growth. Introduce the new food gradually, along with the regular diet.

For two days, replace 25 percent of the regular diet with the new food and mix it thoroughly. For two more days, replace 50 percent of the original diet with the new diet. For the next two days, substitute 75 percent of the regular diet with the new food and mix it well. On the seventh day, feed the new diet exclusively.

Feed your new kitten or adult cat in a very calm, relaxed atmosphere. Subdued lighting and one or no human beings present is best. At some point you will probably want to change your cat's diet based on what is available, what you want to spend, personal preference, and the cat's changing needs. Refer to Chapter Three, ''The Eating Machine,'' for complete information regarding feline nutrition.

A Place to Sleep

The cat bed. All cats, young and old alike, seek out a soft, cozy place to sleep at night and a different one to catnap in during the day. Over the years your new friend will try out every conceivable place that you can think of, and a few that never occurred to you, from your bed to your sofa to your underwear drawer. But he will always return to the one place that has his scent on it and is securely established as his own. That place should have a cat bed in it that you purchased before he arrived.

It can be a simple cardboard box with a blanket in it or a wicker basket packed with a soft pillow. There are so many different kinds of cat beds for sale, that there is hardly room to mention them all. Most cats appreciate one that has a top on it so that it resembles a small cave or den. Tall, carpet-covered poles with enclosed platforms at the top are brilliantly conceived to satisfy everything a cat needs to sleep safely, sharpen his claws, and enjoy a high position in the room. Such cat furniture is pricey but well worth it, considering what it will save in wear and tear of your personal furniture. Try to locate the cat bed in some snug corner, on a higher level than the floor.

Cat Carrier

There will be times, early in the game, when you will have to take your pet from one place to another. A trip to a veterinarian's office, a visit to a friend, or even a weekend drive are all possibilities. To accomplish this you will need a container to place the cat in so that he will be unable to escape from your protection. Placing a cat in a sturdy carrier makes him safer, more comfortable, and less frightened than he would be loose in a car.

There are two styles of cat carriers: the soft kind and the hard kind. A *soft carrier* is similar to an overnight bag, with breathing holes in it. Some have a mesh screen at the bottom for the cat to see out. Others have a plastic window for the same purpose. Adequate ventilation is of the utmost importance. A *hard carrier* resembles a piece of old-fashioned luggage, with a handle at the top making it easy to carry. Most hard carriers have a transparent top made of plastic so the cat can see out and be seen by you. These, too, must be well ventilated with breathing holes surrounding the body of the case.

Do not buy a carrier that is too much larger than the cat's body. Of course large cats require a larger carrier. But cats do not want too much space when they are being transported. A snug area with just enough room to move around in allows for maximum utilization of body heat and comforts the cat. Never use this equipment for shipping your cat by plane or other common carrier. Shipping an animal is a different matter altogether and requires specially designed shipping crates. Each airline has its own standards and requirements and will inform you about them upon request.

Line the bottom of the carrier with a towel or newspaper for comfort, traction, and hygiene. Avoid use during hot and humid weather, if possible. During warm weather cat carriers can bring about heat prostration if they are not properly ventilated. Place a small plastic sack of ice cubes wrapped in a towel in the corner of the carrier during hot weather. This will help avoid this life-threatening condition.

Scratch Post

Every cat needs a scratch post. It is important to have this useful device in the house when your new cat arrives. Part of the introduction to his new home should be a brief lesson on the scratch post. It could save you hundreds of dollars by avoiding damaged furniture, carpets, curtains, clothing, and other possessions. There is more to cat scratching than you might imagine. Refer to Chapter Five, "The Cat Train," for more information about this important subject. It is essential to understand that cats scratch with their claws because of a physical and psychological need to do so. Cats develop behavior patterns early in their lives that are difficult to change. Unless you set the proper pattern of behavior quickly, your cat is going to scratch whatever is handy and appealing. In all likelihood it is your furniture that is going to be damaged. Once the problem begins, it is hard to stop.

Many experienced cat breeders use disposable scratch posts made of corrugated cardboard. This convenient product is usually imbued with catnip and is very appealing to most cats. A cardboard scratch post is a rectangular object, approximately eighteen inches long by six inches wide, that lies flat on any surface. Your cat or kitten should be placed on top of it and allowed to get its scent on it. Hold the front paws and move them up and down along the rough surface, initiating scratching motions that are normal for a cat. Few scratching problems ever develop when this technique is employed early and often.

Most permanent scratch posts are vertical pieces of wood, attached to a flat base and covered with carpet, canvas, or burlap. Cats will use them instead of your furniture *if they are high enough.* A cat must be able to reach the top of it with its front claws when standing on its hind legs. There is nothing more useless than a scratch post that is too short. An effective scratch post can simply be a log lying horizontally or leaning vertically against the wall if it is secured to the floor. Other posts are made of cork or loose fabric of all kinds.

Cat furniture of all sizes, shapes, and types provide some

kind of covering or outer material designed for cats to claw. The more expensive pieces are tall, elaborate treelike structures with carpeted platforms and covered enclosures that form a kind of feline playground. Although they are costly, they are wonderful. Most cats take to them immediately. They are advertised in every cat magazine, available in many pet supply catalogs, and often displayed by vendors at cat shows.

Leash, Collar, Harness, and ID Tag

Leash. If you plan to teach your kitten to walk with you outdoors, you will need a leash to maintain control. A lightweight nylon or leather leash is all that is proper to use. The leash must be strong enough to prevent the cat from getting away from you yet light enough so that it is not an uncomfortable burden. Nylon cat leashes are colorful, lightweight, and almost stringlike in appearance. But they are strong enough to do the job. *Do not use string, twine, rope, or yarn. They are not strong enough.*

Harness. The proper equipment to accompany a leash is a cat harness. These are usually made of lightweight nylon and are most often purchased as a set with a nylon leash. Harnesses are available in figure-eight format, figure-H format, or other formats. Refer to Chapter Five, ''The Cat Train,'' for instructions on using this equipment.

Collar. The only good reason to place a collar on a cat is to attach an ID tag or license to it. Do not hook a leash to a collar for the purpose of walking your cat outdoors or to maintain control over him. You can *never* be sure it will stay around the cat's neck. There is always the danger of it slipping off, no matter how tight you make it. In order to keep it secure around your cat's neck, it must be so tight that it becomes dangerous.

Cats tend to get themselves in trouble with collars. In an effort to get them off their necks, they may hook their claws on them. Athletic cats have been known to hang themselves by the collar on shrubbery, fences, coat hooks, and all manner of protrusions. The best collars are those that have some sort of escape mechanism built into them. These are referred to as *expandable* or *breakaway* collars. The escape mechanism works with elastic inserts or Velcro straps to prevent strangulation.

ID tag. All cats should wear an ID tag, whether they are allowed to go outdoors or not. Proper identification can prevent heartbreak if the cat accidentally gets out and becomes lost. Have an ID tag made up at your local pet supply store. Have your personal information engraved on the metal so it cannot be rubbed away. The tag should have your name and telephone number on it. An excellent adjunct to the ID tag is an identification mark tattooed on the cat's belly. Consult a veterinarian or animal welfare agency for more information about ID tattoos.

Toys

Cat toys are essential for giving your new pet the pleasure of play, diversion, mental stimulation, and growth. Kittens that are held by humans and given toys at an early age develop into intelligent, contented creatures with a zest for living. Toys stimulate and provoke the senses and elicit a cat's instincts for survival.

Play is an important means of exercise for domestic cats because they rarely experience the demands of the wild. Play is in reality a learning and practicing process for stalking, ambushing, and attacking prey animals such as rodents and insects.

The toys most frequently purchased for cats in stores are little felt mice that are advertised as catnip mice. The truth is that most of these items are manufactured outside the United States and do not contain catnip at all. They are sprayed with a scented substance that is of fleeting interest to the cat and filled with chopped plant or tree bark. Still, some cats do enjoy these felt mice, so they are worth a try. There is, however, an incredible variety of cat toys to choose from. Some are very expensive and some are not.

If you attend cat shows, you will find vendors selling many,

many cat toys, including long peacock feathers that offer enticing movement for your cat. Waving the feather before the cat's eyes in a bouncing motion, tickling the nose and feet, all stimulate the hunter in your cat and will divert the animal for quite a while. A string or a rope is a good toy that can be used in the same manner. A hard rubber ball, a large sewing spool, or almost anything that will roll makes an excellent toy. Containers such as cardboard boxes, large pots, paper bags, straw hats, or even wastebaskets appeal to a cat's instinct to practice hiding and escaping. Try placing a Ping-Pong ball inside an empty tissue box and watch what happens. The finest cat toy available, the one that offers the most play, is a simple sheet of paper, crumpled up and tossed across the room.

Catnip

Catnip can be considered nature's chlorophyll cocktail for the feline set. After a cat nibbles on this herbal substance, you can expect it to roll around on the floor, rub its face against your legs, jump straight in the air, leap about, and end in glossy-eyed calm. In some rare cases, cats have become slightly aggressive after a nip of the mint.

Its usual effect is first to stimulate the cat into unusual movements and antics. After ten or fifteen minutes kitty calms down and settles into an easygoing state of gratification. Those who give their cats catnip believe it to be a harmless source of fun and pleasure for their favorite companions. Many veterinarians agree with this view. But it is surprising to discover how few cat owners use catnip or even know much about this interesting plant.

Watching a cat respond to catnip for the first time can be puzzling or even alarming, but concern usually turns to amusement. If a cat responds to catnip, and some do not, the effect is relatively short, ending in a nice, long nap. It is believed that all species of cats, from lions to pussycats, may experience the mood swing effect of catnip. However, not all cats within each species are affected by the plant.

Catnip is a natural herb that some experts believe is one of the two vegetables cats eat. The other is grass. They eat grass and regurgitate it. This helps them clear their throats of hairballs. (Indoor wheat-grass plants meant for cats to eat will have the same effect on indoor cats.) They eat catnip and digest it. It provides chlorophyll for their digestion and also serves as a tonic, or a stimulant for exercise. Catnip is a mood enhancer, providing a physical and emotional good feeling. In the past people used to drink catnip tea and referred to it as *spring tonic*. In fact, catnip wasn't grown for cats until recent times. It was only grown for humans and was used as a medicinal herb, not a drug.

The plant and the animal were not originally brought together by humans. It happened in nature without any help from cat lovers. Catnip growing wild is attractive to free-roaming felines, and they will find the plants and eat them all on their own. Catnip is not native in North America. It was brought here from Asia and Europe. In England it was originally called *the cat's mint* because domestic cats were attracted to the plant, which is a member of the mint family. In England eating something sparingly is to "nip" at it. Hence the name, the cat's nip. It was brought to North America by early settlers and entered their herb gardens for human consumption.

In earlier times, before the pharmaceutical industry, catnip was a popular herbal medicine to aid digestion, generate perspiration (presumably for the cure of colds and flus), and to reduce body heat and high fevers. It was taken as a hot tea by infusing one ounce of catnip with one pint of boiling water. Adults were given two tablespoonfuls of the tea, and children were given two or three teaspoonfuls frequently, to relieve pain and flatulence. Catnip is sometimes misconstrued as a drug for cats, offering some form of narcotic effect. Although some may hold this view, the majority of animal professionals do not.

According to some veterinarians, catnip, in moderation, is a wonderful treat for a cat. Differentiating catnip from drugs, there has never been any report that catnip affects the animals' cells, chromosomes, or internal organs, such as the kidneys or liver, or that the brain cells have been disturbed. The cat becomes normal soon after having a little fun with the catnip. Cats with catnip toys roll with them, kick them, throw them in the air. If the catnip is in the dried flowered form, they roll around in it and take a little bit in their mouths. It appears to be more of an amusement for cats than anything else.

Many experienced cat owners use catnip to induce their pets to use scratch posts, by rubbing it on them. Some breeders believe catnip works as an aphrodisiac and enhances sexual activity. Others believe it is more like a sedative, calming cats that may be hyperactive or emotionally stressed.

First Aid Kit
See Chapter Eight, ''The Sick Cat.''

Comb and Brush
See Chapter Six, ''A Good-Looking Cat.''

THINGS TO DO

Kittenproofing Your Home
The most important aspect of kittenproofing is not allowing your new cat to get out of the house or apartment. There are many dangers outdoors for a young, playful, curious cat. Check for holes, broken doors, faulty screens, or open windows. A two-to-three-inch opening is all it takes for a kitten to squeeze through.

The inside of your home can also have hidden dangers for a young cat. If your kitten falls into water of almost any depth, he has a good chance of drowning. Look around your home and try to prevent such an accident. Swimming pools, toilets, wells, filled bathtubs, washing machines with the door open, sinks, and pails are all dangerous for a kitten or uninitiated cat. Keep your electric clothes dryer closed as well as your microwave oven. Make sure your kitten isn't sleeping in either one of them before turning it on.

Walk around your home and check for dangling cords, wires,

ropes, shade pulls, venetian blind strings, fishing tackle (especially with hooks), vacuum cleaner tubes, TV antenna cables, computer wires, and even leather thongs on pot holders. They all appeal to a young cat to play with. Fold up all excess cords and tape them to a wall or under a table. Bits of yarn, string, and ribbon are easily swallowed and can cause blockages, constipation, stomach ailments and even death.

Electrical cords are especially dangerous. A kitten is likely to strike at a dangling wire and pull down the appliance on top of himself. This can happen with toasters, blenders, food processors, electric frying pans, coffee pots, and juicers. An accident of this kind can cause scalding, electric shock, cuts, contusions, broken limbs, and internal bleeding.

Every household maintains a well-stocked supply of poisons deadly for children and pets. Many household cleaners are poisonous to humans as well as to animals. Small animals and children are especially vulnerable to common poisons because small doses can make them seriously ill. Poisons most available for kittens to get into include lead (as in paints and ceramics), petroleum distillates such as kerosene, detergents, lye, cleansers, mothballs, insecticides, and all medications, including aspirin, sleeping pills, tranquilizers, and various cold remedies. Any form of illicit drugs can be lethal for cats, from marijuana to methadone, from cocaine to glue. Secondary cigarette smoke is also harmful.

The garage and basement of almost any house offers many dangers to a cat. Antifreeze, motor oil, brake fluid, and windshield cleaner can all be toxic to a cat that is allowed to lick them off the floor. Antifreeze in particular has been known to cause sudden death.

Many plants are poisonous to pets and must be considered when bringing a kitten into the house. Refer to Chapter Eight, "The Sick Cat," for more specific information regarding plants. Children must be made aware of the dangers caused by some of their toys. Bicycles, skateboards, rollerblades, and many other toys that roll on wheels are potential hazards. A plastic bag can cause suffocation if a cat becomes entangled in it. Be particularly careful when closing your refrigerator door. Make sure the cat hasn't jumped in without your noticing. Never allow a kitten to be loose when operating any household machinery such as the vacuum cleaner, the lawn mower, or the mechanical weeding machine. Radio-operated garage doors can also present a hazard. The cat can get out, and the door can also catch the cat off-guard and come down on him.

Screen off your fireplace lest your roaming cat attempt to climb up the chimney. Remove your breakables from table surfaces and countertops. Cover the top of your aquarium. Elevate the height of your bird cage. Keep the hamsters and gerbils in secure cages and place them in a room the cat cannot enter. Cover all trash cans. Close all drawers, cupboards, closets, appliances, and medicine cabinets. Sooner or later every cat gets into trouble. Watch yours until he settles down in his new home, and even then, be vigilant.

Get a Vet

As in caring for a child, when your kitten is in pain, your only concern should be to find a way to heal this important member of your family. Whether it's emergency treatment or preventive medicine, the pet owner today knows that the only person to handle it is the animal doctor—the vet. In reality, there is little romance to veterinary medicine. The work is hard, messy, and sometimes heartbreaking. If there is anything attractive about it (beyond best-sellers), it can only be found at the end of a day when an exhausted vet wipes a tired brow and acknowledges having alleviated pain and prevented suffering.

Doctors of veterinary medicine are often expensive, difficult to talk to, behind schedule, and overbooked with appointments. Their waiting rooms are usually as crowded as an ark with cats, dogs, and parakeets tripping over one another while distressed humans hope for the best. Ordinarily, no veterinary waiting room has carpeting (for obvious reasons). Taking your cat to a veterinarian's office is not always a happy experience, unless a life is saved, a wound healed, a misery avoided. Who else can send you and your feline companion home in good health?

Every pet owner sooner or later will require the services of a veterinarian. It is always best to know which one you will be using *before* your cat becomes sick, so choose a veterinarian prior to choosing your pet. It's very important. *Ideally, a kitten should be given a complete medical examination before entering your home and becoming attached to your family.* Some pets have incurable diseases and cannot be kept. There is no experience more wrenching than coming to love a baby cat only to give it up. It is also important to select your veterinarian in advance in case your cat has an emergency situation when there's no time to hunt for a doctor.

Also, if your cat has internal or external parasites, they should be treated by a veterinarian before allowing them to contaminate your home. Parasitic infestation of kittens is very common. You can almost count on it.

What makes a good vet? A good veterinarian is one who stays current with advances in medical science and has some talent for diagnosis. He or she must be a person with an inquiring mind and keen powers of observation. Your vet should like and understand animals. Perhaps equally important is the ability to understand and get along well with people. A good veterinarian has compassion for people and animals in trouble.

How to choose a veterinarian. Because most people find a veterinarian by word of mouth, you should speak to other cat owners and get a consensus of opinion about the ones they use. Price is no small matter and is something you should be able to discuss with any veterinarian. Cleanliness is another major factor. When you enter a vet's office, observe if it is neat and clean and odor-free. Are members of the staff (including the doctor) wearing clean gowns, uniforms, or work clothes? Are the floors swept and mopped? Are animal "accidents" cleaned up quickly?

Experienced cat owners believe you should select a vet that conforms to your needs and is sympathetic with your concerns about your pet. Look for someone who likes cats and who has a competent and caring staff. A veterinarian should keep in touch with caring facilities and learning institutions in order to stay current and continue to learn. He or she should not be afraid to admit, "I don't know, but I'll find out." Communication between a veterinarian and a cat owner is of vital importance. A veterinarian must be able to explain things to a client with patience and clarity and be willing to listen. It is essential to develop a relationship with your kitten's doctor.

In veterinary medicine as in human medicine, a skilled diagnostician is priceless. Luxurious waiting rooms and fancy office furniture have little to do with a doctor's skill. There are those veterinarians who bridge the gap between science and art. Such doctors combine experience with a "sixth sense" to identify an ailment when others cannot. It is only through trial and error that we can find such veterinarians, but they are out there.

Is your veterinarian reasonably able to maintain your cat's health and cure his ailments? Is he or she compassionate? Does he or she answer all your questions? Is medical service available over the weekends and during holidays? Answer these questions and you will know if you have chosen well.

Doctors of veterinary medicine can be found quickly in your Yellow Pages under two headings: *Veterinarians* and *Animal Hospitals*. You can also call your local veterinary medical society for referrals.

Get your new kitten examined. The first thing you should do with your new cat is to have him examined by a veterinarian, even before going home, if possible. It is surprising to discover how many pet owners are unaware of the necessity of a complete annual checkup for cats. During the course of the first physical exam, a complete vaccination program must be initiated. Early immunization helps prevent distemper, hepatitis, leptospirosis, parainfluenza, parvovirus, and rabies. The single most important fact about vaccination is often missed by pet owners: an annual booster shot is required to maintain the animal's immunity.

When your new kitten is taken in for his first examination be certain it includes checking both ears, the nose, mouth, teeth, throat, respiratory system, spine or musculoskeletal system, skin, legs, reproductive system, abdominal cavity, cardiovascular system, and anal area. For more detailed information about the annual checkup see Chapter Eight, "The Sick Cat."

Separate Your New Cat from Other Pets

Make sure the new kitten is going to be separated from other house pets for a while. An older cat and a kitten or an older dog and a kitten will eventually work out the terms of their relationship. However, it could be a traumatizing experience for a new kitten to have to adjust to the curiosity or hostile treatment of an older pet. Give the new pet a chance to adjust to being away from his previous home before subjecting him to the curiosity or hostility of the older pet. Keep other pets away for several days if you can. A wire cage or portable gate can be useful for this purpose.

KITTEN GRAFFITI

A new kitten can turn your home into a subway car in less than a week. It is capable of destroying carpets, upholstery, floors, furniture, and walls by scratching, chewing, playing, mischief-making, and of course, by uncontrolled body eliminations.

You have three options for dealing with this. You can live with it, change your pet's behavior, or preserve your home by kittenproofing it. This is not a course on beautifying the pet place for interior designers. This is about sparing your home the unsightly results of cat and kitten "enthusiasm." It will be especially useful if you are still shopping for a cat. But the patient cat lover can also benefit from this information. It is a matter of decorating with materials and products that can stand up to the potential abuse of normal cat behavior or making some environmental changes.

The most obvious problems are usually found on the floor. On occasion, cats and kittens have housebreaking failures, and also vomiting. This can permanently stain expensive carpeting.

Scrapes and deep scratches are another problem, when cats use the bare floor to exercise their claws. You need a floor that can withstand the worst animal assault and still look good. You can switch to a first-rate wood floor, use permanently waxed vinyl or urethane floor covering (a new and improved form of linoleum), or buy one of the new stain-resistant carpets.

If you decide to go for easy-to-clean wood floors, seriously consider oak (sanded and finished) because it wears well, or prefinished laminated flooring because of its resistance to moisture. Look under your carpet. You may have a decent wood floor that can be restored. A hard finish on your floor, such as polyurethane or shellac, will definitely withstand any abuse your cat can dish out. If given enough time to cure, the finish will resist your pet's digging and scratching.

The best floor covering for pet owners is vinyl or urethane sheets or tiles. Linoleum is being used less and less because its felt backing causes moisture damage and because it does not stand up to serious abrasion. Once upon a time nonporous floor coverings were found only in kitchens or bathrooms. But now the wide selection of sophisticated colors and patterns have made it possible to use them in almost any room of the house.

Sheet vinyl offers the advantage of an almost seamless surface, although vinyl tiles can be installed by anyone, especially if they are self-sticking. All you do is peel off the paper to expose the adhesive, place the tile on the floor, and press down firmly. Such a floor will give you an important advantage when dealing with a cat who insists on coughing up hairballs (in front of dinner guests, of course). Many leading manufacturers of vinyl and urethane floor coverings offer a no-wax feature with stain resistance, gloss retention, and the ability to withstand abrasion. You can't ask for more. Staining will not be permanent with a no-wax vinyl so long as the stain is not allowed to remain on the surface for a long time. Urethane, however, offers a tougher, more scratch-resistant surface than vinyl. Look for a covering that offers both stain and scratch resistance.

For those who cannot live without their wall-to-wall carpet

or room-size rug, there is also an answer. Stain-resistant carpets have made it possible to have your cake and drop it, too. Some carpets are made from fibers with locked-in stain blockers to protect floors from most household stains, including whatever your cat can come up with. Of course you'd be better off selecting tweeds, tone-on-tones, and pebbled textures to help hide dirt and lint. Patterned designs on stain-resistant carpets help enormously.

To avoid furniture stains from your cat or kitten, look for a Scotchguard Fabric Protector label when you buy an upholstered chair or sofa. Applied at the mill, Scotchguard protective coating is your best chance for resisting pet stains. This product is also available on the shelves of supermarkets and hardware stores as a do-it-yourself spray.

Animal hairs and other kinds of cat-related debris on the carpet can be dealt with handily by any one of the new portable vacuum cleaners. Many of them are cordless and lightweight. Watch the litter fly off the floor with these machines, a dream for pet owners. Many cat scratching problems can be solved by getting a piece of plush, carpeted cat furniture. Some of it is not only practical but quite beautiful. There is an enormous selection of scratch posts available for clawing cats, too, from plush to disposable cardboard. Visit a pet supply store or obtain one of several pet supply catalogs offering tons of cat and dog merchandise.

A QUICK COURSE ON CAT BEHAVIOR

The cat has never really been domesticated in the sense that the dog has. Dogs instinctively live in social structures. Humans are substitutes for other members of the dog pack. But cats live a solitary existence in the wild and are not programmed by nature to live with other creatures, cats or human substitutes. It is only through centuries of domestication, adaptation, and human adoration that cats have gone against their instincts to go it alone. Many house cats could easily revert to the wild state and probably survive with a little luck.

Even in domesticity, for the most part, cats live as solitary an existence as circumstances will allow.

Long-enduring relationships between humans and domestic cats develop along lines similar to those between parents and children, or brothers and sisters. The instant a human assumes the responsibility of feeding and caring for a cat, he or she is eliciting a form of immature dependency from the animal. This childlike behavior may remain for as long as the cat is taken care of. But many of the behaviors of physical maturity develop no matter what. All cats will mate and become mothers and fathers if given the opportunity. They will also become proficient hunters if they are returned to a wild state.

We can see in the domestic cat a paradox of behavior. The skill of the solitary hunter produces an adult capable of instant self-sufficiency. The acceptance of loving care produces an eternal kitten. Therefore, our beloved house cats are both independent and dependent at the same time. It may be the only difference between wild and domestic cats other than size. It may also be a bit of their mystery.

Who can deny that the point to living with a cat (or a dog for that matter) is to enjoy the pleasure of the animal's company. Although cats bring a bit of nature into our paved and artificial world, they are more than simply four-legged houseplants. Cats are unique creatures with a genetically programmed set of behaviors and responses. There are several major areas of feline behavior that are most important for the cat owner to understand. They have to do with territory, hunting, eliminating, and mating.

Territory

Cats place greater importance on their homes than on their families. This is one of the traits that make their habits predictable. They like to sleep in several well-chosen, special places, eat in one place exclusively, and even relieve themselves in the same place. Their outdoor exploring is patterned. Once a cat has established himself in his own world, it is extremely upsetting for him to be uprooted from it, even for a vacation. To a cat a territory is a loosely fixed area influenced by time, space, and other creatures. In the wild, territory is essential for survival, as it must provide a sufficient amount of prey animals to hunt and eat plus offer an area in which to mate and then bear offspring. Territory is sometimes inherited, won in combat, or discovered and claimed after it has been abandoned by other animals. Domestic cats find themselves placed in a territory that is not of their own choosing. It is the human home. However, they make a quick adjustment once they discover that the territory is like a fine hotel with good room service and reliable wake-up calls.

Hunting

Cats are the most efficient hunters in nature. They are unsurpassed predators in constant search for their food. Even a well-fed cat will continue to roam about seeking prey; instinct will have it no other way. Birds, rabbits, mice (and their larger cousins) will trigger the instinct in the mildest cat to stalk, pounce, and kill. Most cats are ready to hunt by four months of age if they've been taught how to do it by their mothers. If not, it's anyone's guess if they will chase mice, and if they do, kill them. It is quite common to see a mother cat with a five-week-old litter return to the nest with a freshly caught, live mouse. The point of the exercise is to teach the kittens what a mouse is for and what to do with it. That is why cats present humans with the catch of the day and then seem to play with it. It is their instinct to teach you what to do so that you'll never go hungry. It would appear that humans are sometimes substitute kittens.

Eliminating

When living in the wild, cats take great precautions to avoid detection so that prey animals are not aware of their presence until it is too late. It is also important that their enemies and competitors cannot not find them. To hide their presence they bury their urine and feces every time they must eliminate. The most inexperienced kitten will use a litter pan for his body waste because in all probability it is the only place in the house where he can dig in a gravel-like substance and bury his scent. It has nothing to do with hygiene or pleasing humans. Getting a cat to use a litter pan is simply a matter of repetitiously carrying him to the box and moving his front paws in the gravel so that a behavior pattern is established. When cats do not use their litter pans, it is almost always because they are upset about something or because they are physically ill. For certain purposes, interestingly enough, all cats will use their urine and feces to announce their presence. For example, claiming territory involves "marking" it with body waste. The same is true for finding a breeding partner.

Mating

To the uninitiated, feline sexuality comes as a rude and often disturbing shock. Feline sexual behaviors create the impression of pain, trauma, and uncontrollable body malfunction. It is of the utmost importance for cat owners to understand that neither male nor female cats are sick or in pain when they lock into the extraordinary behaviors associated with the mating process. It only appears that way.

Domestic female cats may have as many as four or more cycles of estrus (heat) throughout the year, unless they become pregnant or are neutered. Male cats will mate at any time of the year if they are stimulated by a female in heat. Cats become capable of mating between six and eighteen months, depending on the breed, the individual cat, the conditions of the environment, and the amount of stimulation from other cats. In the female, estrus lasts between five to eight days, but can range between three to twenty days. Some experts believe mating shortens the duration of the estrus period; others believe it has no bearing on it at all.

A female in heat behaves at first in an unusually affectionate manner, rubbing against furniture, carpeting, and human legs. As estrus progresses, she may emit low and throaty sounds that can be disturbing. They are meant to attract male cats. The male responds by spraying sexually scented urine against walls and vertical objects, and with aggressive behavior toward other cats.

Novice cat owners must become aware of the overpopulation of pets and the fact that there are simply not enough homes for all of them. Allowing cats to mate cannot be justified. Only experienced breeders attempting to improve a line of pure-breed cats should even consider this activity. Cat owners should have all male and female cats surgically altered to avoid adding to the tragic problem of unwanted kittens that will not be able to find homes.

THREE LESSONS
FOR THE FIRST WEEK WITH YOUR NEW KITTEN

Lesson One

Kittens (and the cats they grow into) are nothing at all like puppies (and the dogs *they* grow into). Cats may seem more controllable, but they are not. They go their own way despite their delicate mewing, purring, or rubbing against your legs. First-time cat owners mistakenly believe that kittens are creatures to be dominated and ordered about like dogface soldiers in basic training. Anyone who has ever lived with a cat knows the folly of this. If you attempt to control your new cat like a dictator, he will run from you on sight, perhaps hide for days. Rejection from a kitten can be more upsetting than from a room full of teenagers.

Cats are like politicians. They must be buttered up, handled gently, tempted with tidbits, complimented, and shown the rewards for cooperative behavior. Despite their preference for solitude, cats soon become attached to their families and come to depend on them for food, shelter, and intimacy. *But you must accept this on the cat's terms.* You must patiently wait for the kitten to climb into your lap and ask for your attention. Do not force anything. Just let it happen.

Lesson Two

Kittens should not be interfered with while eating, sleeping, toileting, or playing. These activities are personal and cats prefer to be alone for them. If you interfere, you may bring them to a halt and cause problems for you and your cat. Sometimes a kitten will invite you to play with him, but not always. If the little cat looks bored (not tired), then get in the game. All cats love Ping-Pong balls, peacock feathers, catnip toys, anything that rolls, jingles, clicks, or snaps. Even a crumpled piece of paper, if tossed with style, offers a bit of fun. Pet shops and mail-order pet suppliers offer tons of wonderful cat toys. Stock up.

Lesson Three

Whenever a new cat owner discusses the furry blessed event of the family, the subject of strange nocturnal behavior comes up. It's quite predictable. Some have referred to it as "The Midnight Special," but others have called it "The Midnight Crazies." It has been described like this:

"Late at night, after we've all gone to bed and are in a sound sleep, we hear a sudden crash. It could be a lamp falling over or the trash can tipping to the side. Out of a cloud of dust comes the thundering sound of hoofbeats as the feline night stalker races across the entire house, up one wall and down again. The cat stops high atop the highest point it can climb and lets out a chest-beating *MMRRROWL* at the top of its cat's voice and then begins its run again. Only this time it runs sideways, stops in the middle of the room, leaps straight off the ground, and pounces down with all its might. It goes on for ten minutes. When the dust settles we try to get some sleep . . . unless the cat starts it all over again."

Kittens, young cats, and even some older cats are remarkably playful. This behavior seems to peak in the middle of the night. There is a perfectly logical reason for this, but few seem to know what it is. Those who must clear the wreckage in the morning make wild, humorous guesses about it. As this behavior often begins after use of the litter box, the "Midnight Crazies" could be your cat's statement about the pleasures of life. The activity most certainly has something to do with reaffirming territorial rights. Cats claim territory by marking it with their claws (litter box scratching, scratching the furniture) and vocal proclamations (''*mmrrrowl!*'').

There are several reasons why this behavior is displayed late at night. For practicality's sake—this is when the cat has the run of the house without interference. Of course, it is debatable whether cats do anything for practical reasons. They sleep most of the day and appear to have what can only be described as an overflow of energy at night (after we've gone to bed, of course). According to the German feline behavior researcher Dr. Paul Leyhausen, ''Events almost always happen at night. This is not because the cat is predominantly nocturnal, but rather because the animals dislike being observed and are sensitive to noise and commotion.''

Another irritating nighttime activity is play behavior. Although cats are not truly nocturnal creatures, they are very well equipped for darkness. They see better in dim light than most animals, and their superb hunting skills are greatly assisted by the touch of their ultrasensitive whiskers. It has also been suggested that cats, like owls, recognize ultraviolet rays given off in darkness from the bodies of some animals. Their response to the subtle vibrations caused by prey animals plus their remarkable hearing capacity make cats keen night hunters.

It is all too common for kittens and even grown cats to make a routine out of play rituals in the middle of the night. Play is practice for hunting methods, fighting behavior, escape behavior, and sexual activity, as well as simply exercise and fun. The feline technique for hunting is to stalk and ambush, utilizing maximum energy in an instantaneous rush of bursting effort as the cat pounces on its prey. Domestic kittens habitually use even more energy in play than they would when actually hunting. It is little wonder, then, that their nocturnal behavior tends to keep their families awake. Worse yet, the play can become destructive to possessions and property. Garbage pails, lamp cords, books, magazines, clothing—all should be placed out of harm's way before going to bed.

Excessive nighttime activities occur when the owner does

not play with his or her cat frequently, pays little or no attention
to him, or when the cat has slept all day long. This is especially
true for kittens and young cats with a large spill of unused
energy. The solution to the problem is easy. Provide more
opportunities for a variety of play activities. Tossing a crumpled piece of paper around as if it were a ball can be quite
interesting to a cat. Ping-Pong balls are among the feline
favorites. Play is best when it is between cats and humans. Of
course play should also involve toys that cats can enjoy by
themselves, such as wooden thread spools, balls, and various
kinds of squeak toys.

One way to cope with the playful new kitten is to confine the
animal to one room for the night. The best place is the one
where the food, water, scratch post, and litter pan are located.
The only problem with this is the cat's anxiety. Some kittens
will adjust to being confined in one room alone for the evening,
and some will not. You can choose to confine your kitten in
your bedroom if you do not mind having it on the bed. Of
course you cannot do this for the rest of the cat's life, and
sooner or later you're going to have to experience the "Midnight Crazies."

Within the nocturnal overflow of energy, you can see all
aspects of hunting and prey capture. The "crazies" involve
sudden dashes across the room in a crouched position, stalking,
watching postures, creeping, pouncing, seizing with the teeth,
carrying around and tossing objects away. To the novice cat
owner this is a startling and perplexing set of behaviors. But it
is actually harmless, fascinating, and more often than not, quite
funny, if not outright lovable.

Look at it this way, a pet makes so few demands and its
emotional connection is so direct and innocent, that even the
most alienated cannot resist it. A kitten simply needs to be fed,
given a place to toilet, a soft spot to sleep on, and some direct
loving attention. In exchange it will bring the natural world into
the most artificial environment and restore awareness of the
human being's place in nature. When the pet owner understands this, almost any feline antic, no matter how annoying, is

worth the trouble. Be patient. In a week or two your kitten will settle down and think of new ways to get under your skin. Welcome to the wonderful world of cats. Have faith. It does get wonderful. You may want to pause while eating your soup because there may be paws *in* your soup. If happiness is a warm puppy, then devilish delight is a new kitten . . . and the first week with your baby puss will be a challenge.

CHAPTER THREE

The Eating Machine

Food is serious business to a cat. In the wild much of its behavior, activities, and energy goes into finding a meal, which involves hunting, ambushing, attacking, killing, and eating a prey animal. After killing its prey, the cat must then protect it from other predators that are inclined to steal it out from under. It's a jungle out there!

It may come as a surprise to those who pamper their pets with lavish foods and home-cooked meals that nutrition, simply defined, is just the transformation of food into living tissue within the body. It is nothing more or less. In a natural setting, domestic cats or their larger, more ferocious cousins, lions and tigers and all the rest, do not sit down to a great meal every night. They only eat after a successful hunt and then consume as much as they can, in order to tide themselves over until the next meal is found. This may carry over to our house cats who eat more than they should at each meal if given the opportunity. It is an instinct. That's why it's easy to mistake your cat's ravenous eating behavior for real hunger, and then continually overfeed him. However, all cat behavior is not instinctive. A great deal of the domestic cat's feeding behavior is learned from overindulgent humans who generously offer unrealistic amounts of food to the cats they love and adore.

Feeding your cat from your dinner plate is a bad idea because it is very difficult for you to meet what is known about its nutritional requirements. A cat's nutritional needs are quite different from those of human beings, and it's important for pet owners to understand this. What is also of significant importance is the fact that cats have different nutritional requirements from dogs. Meals meant for humans or dogs are definitely not in the best interests of your cat.

From kittenhood to old age, cats rely totally on their human caretakers to assume full responsibility for their health and well-being. A cat must be fed every day of his life by a devoted and knowledgeable human being. Everyone knows that animals cannot survive without food and water. But proper nutrition goes beyond satisfying hunger and survival. Intelligent feeding affects the quality of life for all pets as well as for those who must feed them.

A cat's entire emotional and physical health is influenced, if not determined, by inherited factors, environmental influences, and nutritional intake. It is impossible to overemphasize the importance of feeding a cat properly from birth to old age. Fortunately, nature has *not* made it difficult for the pet owner and cat fancier to achieve at home what happens in the natural state, thanks to science and industry.

Cats in the wild must hunt to survive. They must continually move about if they are to remain close to their food sources. As solitary creatures, they must trail their prey, attack it, and bring it down. Once it has been killed, the first nutritional element consumed is the blood. Next, cats tear open the stomach and eat the partially digested vegetal matter. Unlike humans, cats instinctively eat what is best for them and consume all of the organs, including the liver, heart, kidneys, lungs, and intestines. The bones are then crushed and eaten along with the marrow. Fatty meats, connective tissue, and lean muscle meat follow in quick succession.

Proteins and minerals are absorbed from the blood, bones, marrow, organs, and muscle meat. The vegetal matter in the stomach supplies vitamins and additional minerals. Fat is supplied by the fatty meat and intestines, along with fatty acids, vitamins, and some carbohydrates. Roughage is provided by hair and other indigestible elements, particularly from the vegetal contents. Cats absorb added vitamins and minerals from exposure to the sun and by drinking water. In the wild they obtain a well-rounded nutritional regimen from the prey animals they eat, and derive all the positive effects possible from their diet, assuming they eat often enough. It is absolutely essential for all cats, including pets, to achieve this same level of nutrition if they are to experience long and healthy lives.

HOW TO FEED YOUR CAT

The two prime questions here are "*What* should I feed my cat?" and *How much of it* should I feed my cat?" A commercially prepared cat food or one formulated at home is *what* one feeds. *How much* depends on many things. For example, a growing kitten eats more food in proportion to his body weight than the average adult cat, due to the accelerated body growth that takes place in the first year of life. A pregnant female, or one that is nursing kittens, also eats more food in proportion to body weight. And then there are cats that live outdoors and are very active. Their nutritional needs can be far greater than the average cat because of the energy consumed by their physical activities. Environment and weather play a great role in determining the quantity a cat must eat. A barnyard cat in Wisconsin may require as much as 90 percent more food per day in the winter than a cat living in a condominium in Florida.

Most cats achieve full growth by their first year. Kittens more than triple their birth weight during the first three weeks of life. There is a rapid growth phase that lasts until twenty-one weeks of age. After that, growth begins to slow down, but does not stop until approximately twelve months. At six months of age, a kitten may look full grown, but its internal organs, muscles, teeth, and hair coat continue to develop until twelve months of age.

Consequently, they require more nutrition per pound of body weight in their first year than they do thereafter. This accelerated nutritional need ends once the adult stage is reached. Owners must be guided by the performance of the diet rather than by how much the kitten eats. Kittens should show steady growth, have glossy coats, and a thin layer of fat beneath the skin. The rate of weight gain depends on the individual cat, its temperament, and its activity. Consult a veterinarian for this information about your own cat. Weigh the cat once a week and maintain a record of its rate of weight gain. This will determine whether the diet is sufficient.

Once the cat has reached twelve months of age, it is an adult and requires a maintenance diet. The most practical method for maintaining a cat is to establish an ideal or desired body weight and then feed a sufficient quantity of a high-quality commercial cat food to maintain that weight. Weekly weighings are required during the time when this quantity is being established. After the appropriate quantity is established, monitor the cat's body weight on a monthly basis. Changes of more than 10 percent from the ideal weight should be accompanied by more or less food fed to the cat. *The proper amount of food is the amount that allows the cat to maintain its ideal body weight on a consistent basis.*

WHAT TO FEED YOUR CAT

High-quality, commercially manufactured cat food is the best ration to give your cat. There is no doubt that a brand-name or premium priced commercial cat food will promote growth, sustain life, and provide a nutritionally balanced diet designed for cats, and that is no small matter.

Commercial Cat Food

Dry, cereal type. Dry cat food is a cereal-based source of nutrition consisting of grains or cereals mixed with combinations of meat, fish, and/or dairy products. The premium brands have added vitamins and minerals, balanced to meet the nutritional requirements of cats.

Dry cat food is the most economical form of commercial food for cats. Because of the high density of the food, the cat owner is not purchasing large amounts of water. The moisture content of dry food is 10 percent. Canned foods contain between 70 and 76 percent moisture, making it necessary to feed a cat larger portions in order to maintain adequate nutrition. Cost, therefore, becomes a consideration. Many cats love to crunch their food, and one of the easiest ways of feeding is to select a top-quality dry-food product, and put in a bowl in a quiet, convenient place, allowing a cat to eat whenever the mood prevails.

Soft-moist cat food. This extremely popular form of commercial cat food comes in various colors and is soft to the touch, yet it does not require refrigeration. It is often made to resemble hamburger, stew meat, or meat granules. Cats tend to be attracted to the look, smell, and taste of it. It is made with many protein sources; it may feature only one as the overall flavoring, such as beef or tuna, or may offer flavor mixtures. This form of pet food is more expensive than dry food, but not as expensive as canned "gourmet" types. It is designed to provide complete nutrition.

Canned cat food. Canned cat food is by far the most popular form of food used to feed house cats. The ingredients consist of some form of protein (most often fish or poultry), along with various grains and vitamins and mineral supplements. These are cooked in the can and preserved through the traditional canning process. In addition to its great taste appeal, it provides a significant quantity of water for cats who usually do not drink as much as they should. Canned cat food consists of almost 75 percent moisture and helps maintain our cat's water balance.

Canned gourmet cat food. Of the canned cat foods, these are the most expensive and, interestingly, the most popular. They appeal to the human desire to indulge their pets. They come in such flavors as kidney, liver, chicken, shrimp, tuna, beef, and in many varieties of these ingredients. This form of commercial food is best when used as part of an overall feeding program.

Commercial Cat Food for Special Needs
Feeding a sick or obese cat. Most of the cat foods you buy at the supermarket or feed store are intended for normal

kittens and average adult cats. While some of these foods are of higher quality than others, their intended use is still the same, which is to nourish a typically healthy pet.

However, when a cat is sick or highly overweight, it becomes necessary to change the regular diet to conform with a veterinarian's therapy. A significant alternative to preparing special formulas at home is a commercially prepared canned or dry food that is obtained from your veterinarian. Although these prescribed diets are available in a maintenance formula, they are also formulated specifically for cats suffering with diabetes, colitis, obesity, food allergies, heart problems, kidney disorders, liver disorders, and many other illnesses. These mixtures require specialized formulations using selected ingredients designed for cats with various ailments. If such food becomes necessary it can only be obtained from a licensed veterinarian.

Homemade Cat Food

The nutrition charts and the accompanying text in the booklet *Nutrient Requirements of Cats,* published by the National Research Council, indicate how difficult and complex it is to formulate at home a perfectly balanced diet for cats. Table scraps are too inconsistent and unbalanced to be of any reliable value to a cat's health in terms of maintenance or growth. Preparing the most expensive foods meant for humans will not necessarily keep your pet in good health if the meals are not formulated to conform to the nutritional requirements of cats. For this reason most homemade diets are the least satisfactory and in some cases the most detrimental to the cat. It takes time, patience, and knowledge to prepare in your kitchen a complete and balanced diet for cats.

To accomplish this, first obtain from the U.S. Department of Agriculture a bulletin, "Nutritive Value of Foods," and determine the nutritional values of the various foods you want to feed your cat. Cross-check them against the various nutrient charts for cats in *Nutrient Requirements of Cats,* published by the National Academy Press. It will then be possible to formulate as many varied meals at home for your cat as you wish. It is easier, however, to simply open a box or a can of high-quality cat food.

HOW TO FEED YOUR CAT

Cats, like humans, need varied types and amounts of food at different times in their lives. The following will provide you with a valuable set of guidelines for providing your cat with optimal nutrition throughout its life.

Kittens

From birth to weaning, which usually means from day one to day twenty-eight, mother's milk is the best source of nourishment for kittens, if the mother cat (the queen) has an ample supply for the entire litter. Important antibodies are present in the mother cat's milk for the first twenty-four to thirty-six hours. This first milk is called *colostrum*. In addition to providing immunities, it also supplies newborn kittens with protein, vitamins, and various nutrients. It is essential that the kittens receive colostrum as soon as possible. If they are orphaned or rejected by the mother for any reason, it is imperative to supply them with milk as quickly as possible if the animals are to live. There are several high-quality milk-substitute products available in pet supply stores for orphaned newborn kittens. It is important to understand that cat milk has a greater quantity of protein and fat than cow milk. For that reason the latter cannot meet the nutritional requirements of kittens.

When nursing an orphaned kitten, bear in mind that the animal needs direct stimulation to help him digest food for the first two weeks of his life. You will have to burp the little cat by gently patting his back and then help him to urinate and defecate by rubbing him on the belly. Normally, the mother cat would do this with her tongue. Follow the directions on the milk-substitute product that apply to the kitten's age. Quantities and feeding times will be indicated. Nursing kittens require four or five feedings a day and receive just under two teaspoons per feeding. These commercial products often come with nipples and bottles.

By four weeks of age the kitten is ready to begin being weaned away from a milk-only diet through the gradual introduction of whole food. For two or three weeks a commercially prepared cereal product for weaning kittens should be introduced. Follow the feeding instructions on the label. Mix the cereal with tepid whole or evaporated milk and feed a small quantity four times a day, between nursing sessions with the mother or scheduled milk-substitute feedings. By the sixth week you may begin introducing small quantities of scraped meat or boiled white fish or chicken.

The growth rate of kittens is accelerated during the first twenty-one weeks. In the first three weeks a kitten's birth weight usually triples. Many cats, however, do not reach full maturity for twelve months or longer.

An eight-week-old kitten, fully weaned, requires approximately four to five ounces of canned food or two ounces of dry food per day. Kittens in this age group should be fed four meals a day—the more mixed the diet, the better. Vary the diet from meal to meal with dry food formulated for kittens, a cooked egg yolk (*no* raw egg white), small quantities of whole milk (provided it does not cause indigestion), strained meats (baby food), cooked white fish, cooked white chicken meat, and a very small quantity of cooked liver.

By five months of age a kitten should be fed approximately six ounces of canned or fresh food, two to four ounces of soft-moist food, or three ounces of dry food—divided into three meals a day. Follow the feeding instructions on the label of your commercial cat food if they are provided.

Three feedings a day are desirable for kittens up to eight months of age. A varied diet should be fed to the average house cat for its entire life. Try to avoid any addictions or fixations to any one type of food. Never try to humanize the cat diet in order to make it more palatable. Human preferences and cat preferences are different, although cats will sometimes eat human foods because of the attention that goes along with it. Every cat is different and only the most general rules apply. To some extent allow the dictates of your cat to determine quantities, feeding schedules, and types of food offered.

Clean, fresh water must be available to the cat at all times. This is important for the entire life of the cat.

Adult Cats

Feed an active, ten-pound adult cat (unneutered) a total of six to twelve ounces of regular canned food; eight to eleven ounces of canned gourmet food; from two to five ounces of soft-moist food; or from three to four ounces of quality dry food. Neutered cats require slightly less amounts. Adult cats require about thirty-six calories of food for every pound of body weight. This will vary from cat to cat. *Remember, the proper amount of food is the amount that allows the cat to maintain its ideal body weight on a consistent basis.*

Adult cats are best maintained with two meals a day, spaced between eight and ten hours apart. This aids digestion and helps to avoid obesity, which tends to make cats passive, inactive, and dull, and may create health problems and lead to shorter life spans. A cat should be introduced to a well-balanced cat food early in its adult life and maintained on that ration consistently.

A diet is balanced when the nutrients in the food are present in the proper relationship to one another. The balance consists of water, protein, fat, carbohydrate, vitamins, and minerals. They must be scientifically formulated if the food is going to promote good health; the balance can be thrown off by the slightest change in any one ingredient. Most premium commercial cat foods are meticulously formulated and labeled as "complete and balanced" for some stage of the cat's life, such as growth, maintenance, and so on. The label may state that the food meets or exceeds the National Research Council (NRC) recommendations for minimum amounts of essential nutrients. Watch for foods that indicate they are meant for supplemental feeding only. That means you must introduce an additional set of nutrients found only in complete and balanced foods.

One of the greatest mistakes made by novice pet owners is feeding cats a food that is formulated and marketed for dogs. Cats need more protein in their diet than dogs and have a much higher fat requirement. The feline body also needs more B-complex vitamins than the dog's, and cats easily absorb iron from meat, while dogs do not.

When feeding canned food, serve it at room temperature to keep the food appealing and digestible. Within the bounds of reason, feed your cat on a regular schedule. Consistent routines, including regular feedings, help keep your pet secure and anxiety-free.

If you are going to introduce human foods to your cat's diet, here are some useful tips. All fish must be cooked before feeding. Most cats like fish, but it can be addictive to the exclusion of all other forms of protein. Be sensible about the quantity given and the frequency with which it is fed. Excessive amounts of canned or fresh fish can bring about an ailment known as steatitis, which can be fatal. Milk is not essential in your cat's diet. However, pregnant or lactating queens do need an added source of calcium. Some cats will drink milk, but most cannot digest it properly because of a lack of necessary enzymes. Diarrhea is usually the result. Other good calcium sources are cheese, yogurt, canned salmon, cottage cheese, collard greens, kale, and turnip greens. Tomato juice is beneficial for acidifying the urine in cats with a predisposition to cystitis. Cooked vegetables offer some vitamins and minerals and are desirable if the cat likes them. A teaspoon of animal fat or butter once a day is beneficial. Do not feed your cat an exclusive diet of liver or other organ meats (raw or cooked) or even large amounts on a random basis. It provides an excess of vitamin A, which adversely affects the bone structure. Raw egg white may cause skin problems.

THE FAT CAT

When your cat is as big as your dog (and you have a big dog), you are losing the battle of the bulge. Jelly-belly cats are as endearing as any other, but they will have more medical problems than animals carrying the proper weight. Fat cats also live shorter lives. If you love your heavyset swain, you must consider reducing his weight as an act of kindness and friendship.

The problem is not *overeating* but *overfeeding*. Most normal, untroubled cats will eat as much food as you put in their dish. They think eating is their job. And most cats do their job very well. We've all seen their mad dance to the tune of the electric can opener.

Unless an animal has a medical problem, fat comes from eating more calories than are needed to grow, reproduce, or function on a daily basis. Obesity is almost always a feeding problem.

Cats grow to their full size in the first year of their lives, creating the need to devour more food at that time than a teenager home from school. This is often misinterpreted by novice pet owners as the animal's normal appetite. In addition, food is offered as a reward and as a gesture of love and affection. For those unfortunate animals food becomes more than nutrition. Eating turns into a habit, an obsession, even an addiction, as well as a means of satisfying the emotional problems of the feeder and the feed-ee.

It is not difficult to tell when your cat is overweight. A sagging paunch, a rotund look, and a puffy face with a lethargic presence are the important signs. More than one eighth of an inch of density covering the rib cage indicates obesity. If you're not sure, ask a veterinarian.

To determine your cat's exact weight, stand on a bathroom scale while holding him. Record the amount; then stand on the scale by yourself. Subtract the second weighing from the first and you will know your cat's exact weight. Assuming your vet has verified that your cat is in good physical condition and has told you how much weight he should lose, you are now prepared to put your cat on a weight-reducing diet.

How to Trim Your Pet's Weight

Prevention is the best cure. The health problems associated with obesity are exacerbated with age. The best approach to weight reduction is good feeding management, which, of course, is best begun as a preventive measure during the younger years of an animal's life. The theory is to feed high-quality food early on and in amounts that make sense. See "How To Feed Your Cat." This helps avoid overfeeding and prevents obesity. Do not feed your cat leftovers from your dinner plate, and avoid between-meal snacks. Use only a pet food that claims to be "complete and balanced," in amounts suggested by the label for cats of normal weight.

For cats that are already obese some veterinarians suggest a 60 percent reduction of the diet. The easiest method is to simply feed your cat less food. Although this seems like an obvious statement, it is not. Once your cat has achieved the ideal weight (determined by a veterinarian), the diet can be normalized. (Do not return to the same amount of food that created the obesity in the first place.)

Although this is a workable therapy, the problem is the cat's unwillingness to cooperate. A hungry cat can find so many ways to drive you crazy that you start opening as many cans as it takes to make him stop complaining. A hungry cat will beg, whine, whimper, and steal food if he can. You would, too, if your food intake were reduced by 60 percent.

An acceptable alternative method is to purchase one of several commercially prepared weight-reduction foods. Some can only be purchased from a veterinarian. The idea is to feed the cat the same quantity of food it normally eats but with fewer calories and less fat content. This works as well as any reducing diet.

Another option is to prepare your own homemade diet food.

The following is a diet that is high in protein, low in fat, and designed to satisfy a cat's hunger but help him to lose weight:

1¼   **pounds pork liver or white chicken meat, cooked and mashed.**
1   **cup cooked rice**
1   **teaspoon corn oil**
1½   **teaspoons dicalcium phosphate or 1 Tums tablet (for calcium/phosphorus balance)**

Combine all ingredients. Divide ration into two feedings a day. Yields 1¾ pounds of food. One pound provides 534 calories.

If your cat's ideal weight is	Feed daily
5 pounds	¼ pound
7–8 pounds	⅓ pound
10 pounds	½ pound

Supplement all diets with a vitamin and mineral formula recommended by your veterinarian.
(Diet created by Mark Morris, Jr., DVM, Ph.D.)

People who overfeed their dogs or cats indulge them out of deep feelings for their animals. They are like loving, doting parents who make the mistake of expressing their feelings with food. A misunderstanding of the meaning of love is often seen in fat cats, fat children, and even in fat spouses. A human cooks his or her own goose, but a pet has it done for him. Unfortunately, love is often blind.

THE ELEMENTS OF GOOD NUTRITION

It is important to understand the various aspects of your cat's nutritional requirements if you are to make sound choices in selecting a good diet. The basic elements of nutrition for a cat are almost the same as for humans. The quantities and proportions are different, and a few of the basic requirements vary between the two species. All mammals, including cats, require water, proteins, fats, carbohydrates, vitamins, and minerals. These are the elements of nutrition that provide energy for the promotion of growth, the maintenance of life, and the possibility of reproduction.

Energy

Cats expend energy in almost every form of body activity. Their energy is obtained from either oxidation of food or the destruction of protein sources from body tissue. The utilization of energy obtained from food is influenced by the type of food consumed, how recent the last feeding was, the quantity of food stored in the body, and the amount of exercise the cat gets.

The energy requirements of cats vary. Size, age, activity, state of health, and the environmental temperature all influence these requirements. The energy requirement of a cat per unit of body weight decreases as the cat's weight increases. This means a small kitten requires more energy per pound of body weight than a large cat. In part this phenomenon is due to the higher ratio of skin surface to body volume in the smaller animal, surface through which the energy can be lost. This is the same principle that enables crushed ice to cool liquids more rapidly than an uncrushed ice cube.

The cat that is restricted to a small apartment or house will use much less energy than a cat that is accustomed to roaming the neighborhood and fields. The lactating queen may use up to three times as much energy during heavy milk production while nursing a large litter as she will use during a non-lactating period. A young kitten uses up to three times as much energy per unit of body weight as does an adult cat that is not very active.

Most cats on a self-feeding (*ad libitum*) diet will consume the quantity of food and thus the calories needed to maintain their body weight; this amount varies from individual to individual. Some cats appear to require less than half as much energy per unit of body weight as others. Normally, it is recommended that 0.5 ounces of dry food for each pound of body weight be provided daily. The quantity of soft-moist food will be slightly more than dry food. If canned foods are fed, the quantity will be approximately 1 to 1.5 ounces for each pound of body weight each day.

Water

Water is the foundation of all living things. No life form can exist without it. Living cells require a continuous supply of water in order to function. Water is the most important nutrient for all animal and plant life. It comprises almost two-thirds of the adult cat body weight and even more of the kitten's. Approximately 75 percent of the weight of muscle is water. Whole blood consists of approximately 80 percent water. Bones, without counting the marrow, contain between 20 and 25 percent water. Tooth enamel, the hardest tissue in the body, contains approximately 3 percent water.

Water is the main component of body fluids, secretions, and excretions. It carries food materials from one part of the body to the other. Water is the solvent for most products of digestion. It holds them in solution and permits them to pass through the intestinal wall, into the bloodstream, for use throughout the body. Water also helps regulate body temperature. Only with a generous intake of water can these bodily tasks be performed with any degree of competency.

Having evolved from a desert environment, the feline body can tolerate dehydration with greater ease than many other mammals, including dogs and humans. Cats have the ability to concentrate their urine to a greater extent, the effect of which is to conserve water within the body. This has its limits, however. Long-term dehydration is life-threatening to cats as well as most other creatures. The tendency to concentrate their urine causes some cats to drink less water than they should. It is thought by some researchers to be part of the cause of blockages that form in the urinary tract.

It is, therefore, vital that all cats have free access to fresh water at all times and be encouraged to drink it. Kittens require more water intake in proportion to their body weight than adult cats. Foods containing high levels of common salt, sodium chloride, increase a cat's need for water. Use them if your cat does not drink sufficient amounts of water. Water pans must be kept clean at all times.

The feline body regulates its own drinking water requirement which is determined by body size and weight, food eaten, environmental temperature, physical exercise, personality, and state of health. Because water cannot be stored in the body as other nutrients are it must be replaced frequently. All mammals can survive longer periods of time without solid food than it can without water.

Water is provided from the following sources: drinking water, moisture found in food, and moisture produced as a product of metabolism. It leaves the body in urine, feces, respiration, lactation, glandular secretions, and body injuries.

Protein

Protein is composed of amino acids, which are used by the body for creating new cells in muscles, bones, and organs. Protein is also the raw material of enzymes that are necessary to the body's chemistry. It composes part of the structure of hormones, which regulate many of the body's daily functions. Antibodies, the cells that fight infection, are also made largely of protein. Protein constitutes at least three-fourths of the body mass of all animals (including humans) and is an essential element in the diet of most life forms.

The most common protein sources are fish, meat, vegetables, and eggs. The amino acid composition of the proteins is influenced by the source of the protein and by food-processing methods.

Egg protein is probably the best-known source of balanced amino acids for cats. Other proteins, from fish, meats, and vegetable sources, available in commercial cat foods, approximate the amino acids found in egg protein. Such better-quality proteins are well digested and absorbed.

A cat food containing 30 to 35 percent protein, about 9 percent fat, and 40 percent carbohydrates can meet the protein requirements for a typical adult cat. (Some research indicates that cats can probably exist without carbohydrates, providing the diet contains sufficient fat and protein.) Although the minimum level of protein found in serviceable commercial diets is approximately 30 percent, the extra 5 percent is recommended since the added protein seems to help increase disease-fighting antibody production. A large excess of protein can be tolerated fairly well by the majority of normal cats. Excess nitrogen is broken away from the protein or amino acid molecules and eliminated through the urine. Most of the remaining excess protein is metabolized as energy in the body or may be converted and stored as fat. While this excess protein may not be harmful to young, normal cats, it may be extremely harmful to cats with liver damage or older cats with impaired circulation. Cats with liver and kidney damage tend to accumulate excess nitrogen in the body, and it is dangerous to feed them an extremely high-protein diet.

When feeding extra meat, fish, or other protein sources to a cat, be certain to cook these foods before adding them to the bowl. Uncooked egg white, for example, contains an anti-biotin enzyme that is harmful to cats. Most fresh fish contains an anti-thiamine enzyme. This can cause a thiamine deficiency, resulting in anorexia (loss of appetite), paralysis, abnormal reflexes, convulsions, and a general breakdown of the nervous system. Cook all fish. Cook all eggs.

Carbohydrates

Carbohydrates include starch, sugars (plant and milk), fibers, gums, and other storage components. A large part of most cat foods is composed of carbohydrates, which usually supply the most inexpensive source of energy. When properly prepared, carbohydrates are well utilized by normal cats.

Carbohydrates are utilized to form glycogen, by which the body stores energy, chiefly in the liver. Excess carbohydrates are converted to fat. A deficiency of carbohydrates is rare because protein and fat are utilized for energy in their absence.

Some sugars (carbohydrates) are efficiently used and tolerated by normal cats. Others, like *milk sugar* or *lactose,* may be poorly utilized by some cats. Many cats cannot synthesize adequate quantities of the enzyme, lactase, required for digestion of the milk sugar. This is particularly true of older cats. When the lactase level is low and milk sugar is high, the milk sugar tends to ferment in the digestive tract and can produce diarrhea. This is why some cats tend to have diarrhea when given too much cow's milk, which is high in lactose. Young kittens fed too much cow's milk may suffer digestive upset for the same reason.

Carbohydrates are thought to be necessary as a source of energy and to regulate water resorption in the lower digestive tract. The amount fed is dependent on the amounts of other nutrients making up the diet, but the maximum carbohydrate content in the diet of an average animal should not exceed 65 percent of the cat's diet (on a dry weight basis).

Fat

Each cell in the body is a source of heat, which in turn produces the energy required to maintain day-to-day existence. This heat requires fuel, which comes from food or nutrients ingested daily. Fat is a concentrated source of energy (or fuel) and supplies over twice as much energy potential as carbohydrates or protein. It supplies essential fatty acids and carries vitamins A, D, E, and K. It also adds to the palatability of food. Fat is easily stored in the body, providing a quick source of energy when needed. A pound of fat contains 4,268 calories ready to go to work if called upon.

Most commercial dry cat foods contain 8 percent or more fat. High fat intake can cause diarrhea. When a cat ingests more calories than it expends, the excess nutrients are converted to fat and stored in the body. This is the principle cause of obesity. It is also important to understand that if an unusually high portion of fat is given to a cat it will satisfy its hunger for calories and cause it to eat less food, thus starving the body of sufficient amounts of required proteins, vitamins, and minerals.

Most fats contain many different kinds of fatty acids. Some

of these have a high melting point; these fatty acids are usually found in the fat from cattle, sheep, and horses. Other fats contain a large quantity of low-melting-point fatty acids, which are mostly semisolid or liquid at household temperatures. These fatty acids are found in the fats of pork and chicken, and in highly unsaturated vegetable fats, such as corn oil. The source of dietary fats determines to some extent the type of fat deposited in the cat's body and the resulting body-fat firmness.

Most fatty acids in cereals are highly unsaturated. Thus some cereal grains are good sources of fatty acids. Fish contain an extremely high proportion of unsaturated fatty acids of a type that oxidizes rapidly and, unless processed with care, can produce a vitamin E deficiency and lead to steatitis (yellow fat disease) in cats. This condition may be precipitated by feeding stale wheat-germ oil, or cod-liver oil or other fish oils that are in the process of going rancid. It can be prevented by supplying adequate vitamin E in the diet, adding antioxidants during processing, carefully controlling the processing of the fish, and avoiding feeding stale or rancid oils.

Fat is a very important aspect of sound nutrition. Many experts agree that fat is beneficial in all cat diets from 8 percent up to 17 percent depending on the age of the animal. There is no doubt that cats love fat and that it is good for them (providing it is the right kind and in correct amounts). Too much fat can be ruinous to the animal's health, just as insufficient fat can be detrimental.

Vitamins

Vitamins are complex organic compounds required in small amounts for normal health and growth. The precise requirements of many of the vitamins for various animals, including humans, are unknown. They are dietary essentials and are accepted as properly proportioned in high-quality "complete and balanced" commercial cat food.

Vitamins are categorized in two groups, depending on their solubility. One group includes *fat-soluble* vitamins (A, D, E, and K), and the other *water-soluble* vitamins, which include

B-complex and C vitamins. Understanding this can help the cat owner understand the nutritional needs of his cat. Some vitamins can be formed within the body from other food nutrients, while others must be present in the diet. Fat-soluble vitamins tend to oxidize (deteriorate) easily. This means that fats becoming rancid, or oxidizing excessively, may be devoid of these vitamins and should not be fed to cats.

The amounts of vitamins needed to meet dietary requirements are small, and many vitamin sources are regularly included in prepared quality cat foods. Consult your veterinarian for detailed information regarding specific cats and their vitamin and mineral requirements.

Vitamin A. Vitamin A is necessary for normal growth, reproduction, maintenance of tissues, hearing, and vision, particularly in dim light. It also helps keep the skin and inner linings of the body healthy and resistant to infection. It occurs only in foods of animal origin. Many vegetables and fruits, particularly the green and yellow ones, contain a substance called carotene that most animals can change into Vitamin A. Cats can utilize vitamin A from chemical or animal sources efficiently.

A deficiency of vitamin A leads to emaciation and tissue malfunction. Large, coarse skin lesions may indicate that the cat is not receiving adequate vitamin A. This may be the result of a deficiency of vitamin A in the ration, or it may be due to a particular cat's inability to absorb the A and/or the fat that is available in the diet. Extra vitamin A can be supplied in the cat's ration and even applied topically to the skin lesions. Since cats lick themselves so much, they may remove the vitamin A from the skin and absorb it internally. Vitamin A can also be absorbed through the skin in some circumstances, although this is an inefficient route. Others signs of vitamin A deficiency include loss of appetite, poor growth, skin lesions, dryness, scaling, scratching, and weak and affected eyes. A severe, prolonged deficiency may aggravate respiratory infections and can be fatal to the cat.

Liver is an outstanding source of vitamin A. Significant

amounts also are found in eggs, butter, whole milk, and cheese made with whole milk.

Vitamin D. Vitamin D is important in building strong bones and teeth, because it enables the body to use calcium and phosphorus. It is primarily associated with calcium absorption, transportation, and deposition within the body. Kittens on a diet with an imbalanced calcium-to-phosphorus ratio and inadequate vitamin D are susceptible to rickets. Vitamin D requirements are reportedly much lower for adult cats, and there appears to be more danger of overdoing with vitamin D than of deficiencies.

Calcium absorption from the digestive tract is influenced by the amount of vitamin D in the cat's diet, the dietary fat level, and body stores of vitamin D. Vitamin D is necessary for the effective passage of calcium across or through the intestinal wall and into the bloodstream. This nutrient may be produced by the sun's radiation acting on the fat content of the skin. The cat can produce vitamin D efficiently by this route, although it has not been fully confirmed. Vitamin D_3 from animal sources and vitamin D_2 from irradiated plant sterols are both effectively utilized by the cat.

A severe vitamin D deficiency will prevent normal calcification of the bones of cats even when ample calcium is present, resulting in rickets, irregular teeth, and other skeletal defects. An excess of vitamin D may cause calcium to be deposited in large quantities in the heart, lungs, muscles, and blood vessels. An extreme excess of vitamin D can kill animals.

Few foods contain much vitamin D naturally. Milk with vitamin D added is a practical source if your cat is one who can tolerate it. Small amounts of vitamin D are present in egg yolk, butter, and liver. Larger amounts occur in sardines, salmon, herring, and tuna. Direct sunlight is another source.

Vitamin K. Vitamin K is considered the anti-hemorrhagic (anti-bleeding) vitamin. Under normal conditions it is synthesized in the intestinal tract of cats and other animals. When certain drugs are given or when specific stress occurs, vitamin K may not be produced in quantities sufficient for normal requirements. This is why vitamin K (menadione bisulfite) is added to commercial cat foods. When bacteriostats are administered orally or included in the diet, added vitamin K is warranted. Like other fat-soluble vitamins (A, D, and E), K requires fat intake and bile salts in order to be absorbed and utilized. Vitamin K is found in green vegetables and is also synthesized by bacteria in the intestine. Consult a veterinarian before giving vitamin K supplements to your cat.

Vitamin E. In human nutrition vitamin E is one of the more controversial issues. Many have claimed that vitamin E can promote physical endurance, enhance sexual potency, prevent heart attacks, protect against air pollution, and slow the aging process. Discovered about fifty years ago, the vitamin has also been described as a cure, preventive, or treatment of cancer, muscular dystrophy, ulcers, burns, and skin disorders. The dangers of promoting vitamin supplementation lies in its use as a substitute for *medical* therapies for already existing illnesses. Vitamin E, as a matter of accepted medical opinion, should be taken only as a preventive against vitamin E deficiency. If it is to be used as a medical therapy, it is recommended that a veterinarian be consulted first. Approximately fifty international units of vitamin E per kilogram of food is usually recommended as a minimum for cats.

Vitamin E is a biological anti-oxidant and is considered necessary for several body functions. It is called the "anti-sterility" vitamin because in cases of vitamin E deficiency, the ovum becomes fertilized but fails to become implanted in the uterus. The developing embryo may either die of "starvation" or just pass out of the tract. Too often, vitamin E is destroyed in the body by feeding wheat-germ oil, cod-liver oil, or other fish oil that is going or has gone rancid.

Muscular and nerve degeneration resulting from steatitis (yellow fat disease), which in turn is associated with a vitamin E deficiency, has been described in cats and mink. In the acute phase, steatitis is characterized by a general soreness, anorexia (loss of appetite), depression, signs of pain, and constant elevated temperatures of 104°F to 105°F. Neutrophilia (an increase in the white cell count of the blood) is common. Body fat on biopsy is generally found to be firm and light yellow to dark brown in color.

Fats in the process of becoming rancid apparently destroy vitamin E in the ration and in the animal's body. If wheat-germ oil or other unsaturated fats or oils must be fed by the cat owner, these oils should be kept in the refrigerator after the container has been opened, in order to retard oxidative rancidity. Any such oil that you even remotely suspect to be stale should be discarded.

One reason little is known about vitamin E is that E deficiency is almost impossible to produce in human subjects. To withdraw all sources of vitamin E is almost to withdraw food itself, since the vitamin is present to some extent in most foods and in large amounts in vegetable fats and oils. The major sources of vitamin E are unrefined soybean, cottonseed, and corn oils; wheat germ; whole grains; and nuts. It is also found in smaller quantities in green vegetables, beans, and eggs.

Biotin. Biotin is generally thought to be produced by intestinal synthesis in normal cats. In cats with miliary eczema (small skin lesions), English researchers have indicated that dietary biotin has produced eczema remission and improved hair coats.

Biotin is inactivated by an enzyme, avidin, in raw egg white. This is the main reason that raw eggs should not be fed to cats, since they might produce a biotin deficiency. Simply cook all eggs before feeding. Biotin is found in many foods, including egg yolk, milk, liver, and yeast.

Thiamine (B_1). The cat has an unusually high requirement for thiamine. Some of the thiamine in canned cat foods is destroyed by processing. In addition, some raw fish contain an enzyme, thiaminase, that inactivates thiamine. When a thiamine deficiency is suspected, the daily dosage should be 1.6 mg per 100 gm dry diet consumed. Although cooking destroys thiaminase in fish, this enzyme may already have destroyed the thiamine that once was present. Therefore, fish is an unreliable source of thiamine.

Thiamine helps convert glucose into energy or fat. When thiamine is reduced in the cat's body, the animal's energy level is seriously diminished. Thiamine deficiencies in cats produce anorexia (appetite loss), vomiting, weight loss, dehydration, paralysis, prostration, abnormal reflexes, convulsions, and cardiac disorders.

Extra carbohydrates, such as bread and potatoes, and extra exercise, increase the cat's requirements for thiamine. The need for thiamine is decreased slightly when higher levels of fat are added; thus, composition of the diet influences the vitamin requirement.

Sources of thiamine include whole grains (especially wheat germ and rice bran and polishings), brewer's yeast, pork, milk, nuts, liver, peas, soybeans, and most dried beans.

Riboflavin (B₂). Riboflavin is one of three B vitamins (thiamine, riboflavin, and niacin) that play a central role in the release of energy from food. They also help promote proper functioning of nerves, normal appetite, good digestion, and healthy skin.

Riboflavin is used in many body processes, especially those involving healthy skin, eyes, and the linings of the mouth and digestive tract. If a deficiency of riboflavin occurs, cats will develop anorexia (appetite loss), with a resulting emaciation that, unless riboflavin is again supplied, will lead to death. Loss of hair around and on the head sometimes occurs in riboflavin deficiencies, and cataracts have been observed in some deficiency experiments. In the domestic setting, however, deficiency does not occur in ordinary diets and is only encountered in abnormal situations, where the cat has been severely deprived, coupled with a heavy demand for riboflavin, as in lactation or infection during the growth period.

The daily requirement of riboflavin lies between 0.15 and 2 mg according to the diet and metabolic demands. The principal sources of riboflavin are liver, brewer's yeast, and milk. Whole grains and green vegetables are also good sources of this nutrient. If the greens are cooked, the water-soluble vitamins will leach into the cooking water, which should therefore be fed along with the vegetables.

Niacin (B_3). Signs indicating a deficiency of niacin include inflammation of the skin, loss of appetite, ulcers, and other abnormalities, including diarrhea, emaciation, and redness of the buccal (cheek) cavity. Severe deficiency can be fatal. Unlike most other animals, the cat does not have the ability to convert the amino acid tryptophan into niacin. Since niacin is available in commercial cat foods and stable in the diet, there is almost no opportunity to see a true niacin deficiency when modern commercial rations are provided.

Niacin sources include brewer's yeast, wheat germ, liver, and kidney. Whole grains, fish, eggs, meat, and nuts are also good sources.

Pyridoxine (B_6). Pyridoxine is one of several co-enzymes that help metabolize amino acids. This vitamin also helps make possible the utilization of carbohydrates in the body. In animals with a pyridoxine deficiency, slow growth, convulsions, and hyperexcitability are produced. Kidney lesions and the formation of oxalate calculi (stones in the bladder, urethra, or kidneys) have been associated with a vitamin B_6 deficiency. The best sources of pyridoxine are meat, egg yolks, liver, whole grains, brewer's yeast, heart, and blackstrap molasses. Canning, exposure to light, and excessive storage time tend to destroy its potency.

Pantothenic acid. A deficiency of pantothenic acid is accompanied by weight loss, fatty deposits in the liver, and disturbances of metabolism. The modern pet owner will probably never observe a deficiency of pantothenic acid, since it is available in commercial cat foods, is stable, and is also synthesized to some extent in the digestive tract.

Excellent pantothenic acid sources are brewer's yeast, liver, kidney, heart, wheat germ, and whole grains.

Choline. This nutrient, which is part of the B complex, is important in the metabolizing of fats and in many biochemical reactions. Choline deficiency in cats has been characterized by weight loss, fatty deposits in the liver, and hypoalbuminemia (an abnormally low concentration of certain proteins in the blood). Choline is obtained from liver, kidney, wheat germ, brewer's yeast, and egg yolk.

Vitamin B_{12} (Cyanocobalamin). Vitamin B_{12} is essential for the function of all cells in the body, but especially for bone marrow, the central nervous system, and the intestinal tract. It is retained in the liver and kidneys and is important in metabolizing nucleic acids and folic acid. Vitamin B_{12} is of primary importance in red blood cell formation. It is essential to the prevention and cure of some types of anemia and is necessary for the development of healthy kittens. The precise level of vitamin B_{12} required by cats is not known. However, the synthesis of vitamin B_{12} by intestinal bacteria, combined with the B_{12} found in cat foods, helps ensure that a deficiency will not occur. Vitamin B_{12} is found in whole grains, meat, fish, yeast, and liver.

Vitamin C. Vitamin C is another of the controversial elements of nutrition, with ideas conflicting on the subject. From *Nutrient Requirements of Cats* (National Research Council, 1986): "Ascorbic Acid [Vitamin C]—Repeated trials have failed to demonstrate a need for dietary ascorbic acid in cats (Carvalho da Silva, 1950). Successful growth and reproduction are routinely obtained with commercial and purified (Kang, Morris, and Rogers, personal communication, 1985) diets containing no supplemental ascorbic acid."

From *The Cornell Book of Cats* (Cornell Feline Health Center, 1990): "Vitamin C (ascorbic acid). Cats normally synthesize vitamin C from glucose, so there is no need to supplement the diet. (An exception is made in the case of severe infection, which may impair the body's ability to synthesize vitamin C. In such cases, supplements should be given.) Vitamin C is sometimes recommended as a means of acidifying the urine to prevent *feline urologic syndrome.* Since Vitamin C is water-soluble and rapidly excreted in the urine, it must be given five to six times daily to be effective, which makes it impractical as a urine acidifier."

This very essential nutrient was traditionally thought to be manufactured or synthesized within the tissues of cats. However, some experts feel there are individual differences among cats and that it is impossible to know which cats create their vitamin C and which do not, or if it is being synthesized in adequate quantities.

Vitamin C helps create collagen, a gelatinous material that helps hold the body's cells in place. It also assists in normal tooth and bone formation and aids in healing wounds. Probably the most controversial questions about vitamin C concern its role in aiding the body's immune system. The controversy centers on the effectiveness of vitamin C as a therapy for the common cold, cancer, and other diseases. Vitamin C (ascorbic acid) occurs naturally in citrus fruits, strawberries, cantaloupe, watermelon, tomatoes (tomato juice), broccoli, Brussels sprouts, cabbage, cauliflower, green peppers and some dark-green leafy vegetables such as collards, kale, mustard greens, spinach, and turnip greens, in addition to potatoes and sweet potatoes, especially when baked in the jacket.

Minerals

Minerals are very necessary in the cat's diet and enter practically every phase of body activity. Cats would not live very long with a mineral-free diet. Minerals maintain the acid-base balance within the body and help regulate most body activities.

Because of their interrelationships, minerals should always be considered as a group and never as separate entities. Their requirements and proper ratio are affected by a change in any one. If large doses of calcium are given improperly, for example, a diet which is adequate in all trace minerals may become deficient in some. It is for this reason that vitamin and mineral supplementation requires professional advice.

Minerals are essential for preserving acid-base balance, tissue structure, and osmotic pressure (fluid movement within the body), as well as constituting essential components of various enzyme systems. Some minerals, although important for maintaining good health, may be harmful when larger-than-necessary amounts are given. Such is the case with the calcium/phosphorus ratio.

Calcium and phosphorus must always be discussed together because of the interrelationship between the two. When a deficiency or imbalance between them occurs, poor bone growth or maintenance results. Calcium is the most abundant mineral element in the body. Most of the body's calcium is found in bones and teeth. Combined with phosphorus in an exact ratio it is largely responsible for the hardness of these structures.

The small amount of calcium in other body tissues and fluids aids in the proper functioning of the heart, muscles, and nerves, and helps the blood coagulate during bleeding. Bone formation seems to be optimum when the levels of calcium and phosphorus are adequate and when such associated nutrients as magnesium, vitamin D, choline, fluorine, and manganese are present in adequate and balanced quantities. A large excess of calcium can produce a phosphorus deficiency, and conversely, a large excess of phosphorus can produce a calcium deficiency.

Some foods have a very poor calcium-phosphorus balance. Lean meat contains approximately 0.1 percent calcium and 0.18 percent phosphorus. The proper ratio of minerals is extremely important. But there is none more critical than the calcium-phosphorus ratio. The ratio should remain at *approximately* 1 part calcium to 1 part phosphorus. If a cat owner wants to add lean meat to the cat's diet, the meat should be supplemented with a good commercial diet that can contribute the needed calcium. Calcium or calcium-and-phosphorus supplements should be added to a cat's ration only in carefully controlled quantities. Any such supplementation should not include vitamin D, since this combination, under some conditions, causes hypercalcemia (too much calcium in the blood, possibly leading to calcium deposits in body tissues). It is a good policy to consult your veterinarian before supplementing your cat's diet, especially with a calcium-phosphorus supplement.

Other minerals that have been established as essential to good feline health are magnesium, potassium, sodium and chloride, iron and copper, iodine, zinc, manganese, cobalt, and selenium.

There is no published data on the requirements for cats of sulfur, fluorine, molybdenum, tin, silicon, nickel, vanadium, and chromium, although a physiological need for these elements has been demonstrated in other species.

CHAPTER FOUR

Your Cat's Incredible Body

Your cat is not just another pretty face. Ten pounds of feline gets you 290 bones and tendons, 30 teeth, hundreds of muscles, 4 paws, a tail, and many surprises. A cat is one of nature's supreme achievements. Its elegant body is a masterwork of precision.

It is extraordinary that such a deluxe creature is a commonplace presence in our world at this time. In other times and places, only royalty was privileged to own a cat. Commoners would forfeit their lives for daring to possess one of these creatures that were considered to be gods. Today, almost everyone owns a cat and thinks little of it. To fully appreciate these remarkable creatures one should take a closer look at them. Consider the cat's extraordinary body. It is lithe, graceful, muscular, beautifully proportioned, and capable of doing remarkable things. While the soul of the cat may be a mystery, the body is not.

THE BODY

The feline body, which is to say the frame, can be classified into five types: *tubular, semi-tubular, strong-and-muscular, semi-cobby,* and *cobby.* Body types are based on the shape, length, and breadth of the trunk. When a judge at a cat show handles a cat, his or her hands record the size and shape of the bone structure, the muscle tone, and the basic conformation.

At one end of the spectrum of body types is the *cobby* and

at the other end is the *tubular*. The other body types are variations of the two extremes.

The *tubular* type (also known as *foreign, oriental* or *svelte*) is a body that is medium to long, fine-boned, narrow, and with firm muscles. Breeds of this type are the Siamese, Colorpoint Shorthair, Oriental Shorthair, Balinese, and Javanese.

Semi-tubular refers to a range of body types that are closer to tubular than cobby but varied in length, breadth, and shape. These types can be long to medium-long, lithe, slender but not tubular, muscular, and somewhat broad-chested. Breeds within this classification are the Abyssinian, American Curl, Cornish Rex, Devon Rex, Havana Brown, Japanese Bobtail, Russian Blue, Somali, Singapura, Tonkinese, and Turkish Angora.

Strong-and-muscular cats are solidly built, powerful, muscular with well-developed shoulders and hindquarters, medium to large in length, somewhat stocky, neither tubular nor cobby, deep-chested, and strong-boned. Breeds of this body type are the American Shorthair (rectangular-shaped), American Wirehair, British Shorthair, Chartreux, and Maine Coon Cat (rectangular-shaped).

Semi-cobby refers to a body type with a broad chest and sturdy bone structure that is hard-bodied and muscular, unexpectedly heavy, powerful-looking, firm, and well padded. Breeds of this body type are the Cymric (compact), Korat, Manx (compact), and Scottish Fold.

Cobby is probably derived from *cob*, which is defined as "a short-legged, thick-set horse" or "a male swan." Among serious cat breeders, exhibitors, and show judges cobby is a body type of medium size, heavy-boned, short-legged, broad and deep through the chest, massive across the shoulders and rump, muscular, rounded but with firm muscle tone. The most representative breed of this body is the Persian. Other cobby breeds are the Exotic Shorthair, Bombay, and Burmese.

THE COAT

For some the cat's magnificent hair coat is its most attractive feature. It is, of course, simply a covering of hair. The hair coat consists of three types of hair: primary or guard hairs within the outer coat; awn hairs (intermediate-size hairs forming part of the primary coat); and secondary hairs (downy hair found in the undercoat). *Guard* hairs are thick, straight hairs that insulate the body, protect the skin, and support the sense of touch. *Awn* hairs are thinner and also insulate and protect the body. The thin *secondary* hairs help to regulate the temperature of the body by preventing excessive heat loss. Each hair is attached to an *arrector pili* muscle. When this muscle contracts the hair stands erect. This happens prior to combat (even as play behavior) or as a response to emotional stress.

The hair coat is seen in a wide variety of colors and patterns. Its length can be long, medium, or short, and it is usually straight. The curly (Rex coat) or wirehaired coats are mutations identified with only a few breeds: Devon Rex, Cornish Rex, and American Wirehair.

Coat Types

Pure-breed cats are seen in many coat types. Color, length, and texture of the coat have more influence on the selection of a breed than any other visual aspect of the cat. The feline coat is its primary aesthetic attraction. Many consider the cat's fur to be the most glamorous part of its body. Although show cats are divided into Longhair Breeds and Shorthair Breeds, there are some variations within those two categories.

Hairless cats. Although no cat is totally hairless, the Sphinx, an extremely rare breed, comes closest. The cat is not bald. Thin, short hairs grow tightly packed on its ears, muzzle, and tail. It has no whiskers or eyebrows.

Shorthair cats. Shorthair cats may have a single or double coat. Single coats should look polished and satiny. Double coats should appear thick, full, and plush. A single coat is usually a fine (sometimes silky, sometimes glossy) fur that clings close to the body and is found on such breeds as Siamese, Bombay, Burmese, and Oriental Shorthair. A double coat consists of long guard hairs that display the primary coat color and a thick, downy undercoat, most of which grows on the bottom of the torso. Some of the Shorthair breeds with double coats are Chartreux, Manx, Russian Blue, and American Shorthair.

There are two unusual variations of shorthair coats. They are the *wirehair coat* and the *curly* or *Rex coat*. Both coat types were the result of spontaneous mutations in kitten litters, which were then carefully nurtured for generations into stabilized, established breeds. The wirehair coat can be seen in the American Wirehair, which is similar to the American Shorthair except for its springy, tight, and bent-over fur. The curly or Rex coat is allowed only in two separate breeds by the Cat Fanciers' Association (CFA). They are the Cornish Rex and the Devon Rex. Although similar in type, the Cornish Rex coat has no guard hairs and greater density than the coat of the Devon Rex. It curls, waves, or ripples. The coat of the Devon Rex is also wavy, but it is longer, with less density, than the Cornish.

Longhair cats. The length of the coat of longhair cats varies from two to six inches, depending upon the breed and the part of the body. For example, Persians have long, thick coats of fine texture that fall away from the body. The ruff (similar to the mane on a lion) is substantial and flows from behind the head into a frill along the chest and between the front legs. Some longhair breeds, such as Persians, have a double coat.

Another type of longhair coat belongs to the Turkish Angora. Its coat is medium long on the body and longer at the ruff. The tail has a full brush (plume-like or bushy). Its fur is silky, with a wavy tendency, and is very fine, with a satiny sheen.

The Somali's longhair coat is somewhat different. It is of medium length except on the shoulders, where it is slightly shorter. The breed is double-coated, which means it has a thick, short undercoat, with a topcoat of long hair that is, in the case of the Somali, extremely fine and soft to the touch. Yet another type of longhair coat can be found on the Maine Coon Cat. Its coat is heavy and shaggy, shorter on the shoulders and longer on the stomach and britches (haunches). It has a frontal ruff but not as pronouncedly as on the Persian. Its lengthy tail sustains long and flowing fur. Hair texture is silky and smooth.

Coat Patterns

Tabby Patterns. There are five accepted tabby coat patterns: *Classic, Mackerel, Patched, Spotted,* and *Ticked.*

Classic Tabby refers to dense, clearly defined markings on the body that are darker than the ground color. They are unbroken on top and swirled on the sides, with rings on the tail and bars on the legs. The face is barred with upward pointing lines forming the letter M on the forehead.

Mackerel Tabby refers to dense, clearly defined vertical stripes going around the body. The stripes are narrower than those of the Classic Tabby. The legs are striped with bracelets; the tail is barred. The head is also barred, forming the letter M on the forehead. In some examples of this pattern, the stripes resemble those of a tiger.

The *Patched Tabby* or *Torbie Pattern* refers to a tabby pattern with patches of red or cream.

Spotted Tabby refers to broken stripes appearing as spots.

Ticked Tabby refers to various bands of color on each hair.

Tabby patterns come in prescribed colors depending on specific breed standards, which include Blue-Patched Tabby, Blue Tabby, Brown-Patched Tabby, Brown Tabby, Cameo Tabby, Cream Tabby, Patched Tabby and White, Red Tabby, Silver-Patched Tabby, Silver Tabby, and Tabby and White.

Self. The self coat pattern is a solid color. Each hair is consistently the same color from its tip to its root and is the same on all parts of the body.

Tipped or Tipping. The tipped coat is one that has contrasting colors at the hair ends. Lightly tipped cats are referred to as *Chinchillas,* medium-tipped cats are referred to as *Shaded,* and heavily tipped cats are *Smokes.*

Van (Piebald). This is an almost white coat with patches of color on the head, tail, or legs.

Bi-Color. Bi-color is a solid-color coat with patches of white.

Parti-Color. Parti-color is a coat pattern with two separate colors.

Tortoiseshell. This represents a black coat color with solid patches of red (orange) and cream. It is referred to as a "tortie." If the Tortoiseshell coat has Tabby patching, it is referred to as a "torbie."

Calico. The Calico pattern is a white coat with unbrindled patches of black and red (orange).

Cameo. The Cameo pattern has a white undercoat with red hair tips.

THE WHISKERS

The whiskers are pressure-sensitive hairs or *vibrissae*. When relaxed, they are held sideways. When the cat is concentrated on something, the whiskers are extended forward. It is thought that they aid the sense of touch, much like fingertips, and may be sensitive to air currents, which supply the cat additional information.

THE EYES

For many, the eyes of any cat are the most striking feature, and perhaps the most beautiful. For those who really understand these creatures, feline eyes are more extraordinary for their special abilities than their good looks. The eyes of the cat are dramatically large and reflect how important vision is for these animals. In daylight cats possess about the same visual sharpness as humans. However, cats have about six times the sensitivity of humans to low light levels, allowing their eyes to adjust to sudden darkness faster than ours.

Inside and to the rear of the eye is the retina, which receives light and sends it to the brain as vision. Behind it is a layer of cells known as the *tapetum lucidum*. Its function is to reflect any light not absorbed during its first passage through the retina. This second pass of low light allows cats to see clearly in near darkness, which is when Grimalkin usually goes on the hunt for it prey. Incidentally, when you see your cat's eyes glow in the dark, it is the reflection of light striking the iridescent cells of the *tapetum lucidum.*

Each eye is covered by an upper and lower eyelid. There is also a third eyelid commonly called the *haw.* It protects the eye by sliding horizontally across the surface when the eye is closed, which is why we rarely see it. When not covering the lens, it is at rest within the inner corner of the eye, near the nose.

THE NOSE

Although the nose is part of the respiratory system, it also houses the olfactory nerves providing the sense of smell. The sense of smell is an important tool for protection and influences a cat's appetite and many aspects of its behavior. Cats can smell better than humans but not as well as dogs.

THE EARS

The cat's ability to hear is far superior to the hearing of humans, even that of young children. The highest hearing range for humans is twenty kilocycles. Cats can hear between fifty to sixty kilocycles. They are capable of capturing sounds from the environment that humans are never aware of. They can hear the distant movement and vocal squeaks of mice and isolate them from other sounds. This may explain why they often ignore humans when we speak to them. They may simply be distracted.

THE TONGUE

The tongue is an important part of the mouth apparatus and plays a vital role in eating and personal grooming. It is long, thin, and facile, with an abrasive surface consisting of a group of large papillae (nipple-like projections) which point backward on the upper surface. The tongue serves as a scraping-scooping instrument for eating and as a cleaning tool for the hair coat. It is one of the unique features of the feline body.

THE TEETH

Each half of the jaw, lower and upper, contains small cutting teeth (incisors) and sword-shaped, powerful canines. In addition, cats have three premolars and one molar on each side of the upper jaw, and two premolars and one molar on each side of the lower jaw. Cats bite with the side of their mouths, not with the front. The front teeth, supported by the rough tongue, scrape meat from bones. Cats' thirty teeth are designed for stabbing, slicing, and biting. It is this unique aspect that enables these remarkable creatures to be the most skilled predators in nature.

PAWS AND CLAWS

Next to the teeth, the paws, housing the blade-like claws, are the cat's most important weapons. They are also designed for digging and for traction. The claws are pulled up behind the toes (retracted) as the cat walks and are drawn out like swords when it attacks. When the claws are relaxed, two pairs of elastic bands pull up the first element of each toe. The claws, which are attached to these elements, are then retracted inside a sheathlike fold of skin.

Each front paw has five claws and five toe pads, plus two pads placed higher on the leg. Each rear paw has four claws and four pads, plus a large metatarsal pad. The thick, fatty toe pads cushion shock caused by movement, like well-designed running shoes. They are named according to which bones they protect, such as the *digital, metacarpal, carpal* (front only), and *metatarsal* (rear only). All cats walk on their toes. The pads distribute body weight equally, contributing to the graceful motion that is so notably feline.

THE TAIL

The long and graceful tail is thought to give the cat's body balance when it is running and jumping and to act as a communication signal for its emotions and pending actions.

CHAPTER FIVE

The Cat Train

When the cat's got your tongue, it's usually because he's done some unspeakable thing like ambushed your ankles, attacked your new furniture, or decided the carpet was more to his liking than his cat box. How do you turn a feline imp into a good cat? More to the point, can cats be trained? Yes they can.

It is essential, however, to understand the limitations of cat training. Whereas a dog will learn to heel, sit, come, lie down, roll over, stay, and to respond to various other commands, cats barely do what you want—and on a limited basis only. They do not crave your approval, or get delirious over being told "That's a good boy!" They are an independent species with an ingenious problem-solving ability and in some respects more clever than dogs. They will allow themselves to be taught a few things if there is some advantage pertaining to food or other tangible reward.

Training a cat is based on his predictable behavior patterns and minor vices. By knowing what pleases your cat, you can develop his responses to your commands through food and affection bribery. If you smear a little butter on his paws, he can be distracted from anything; a commercial cat snack will certainly get his attention; give him a cheese omelet and he'll follow you anywhere.

The most important training for cats consists of teaching them to respond to their names, to come when called, to accept housebreaking (cat-box use), and to stop what they are doing when you give the command "No!" All the rest are parlor tricks that may be amusing but have no practical purpose.

WHAT'S IN A NAME?

When Shakespeare wrote, "What's in a name? That which we call a rose by any other name would smell as sweet," he didn't have cats in mind. Cats are smarter than most people think. Once a cat knows his name, he understands that it pertains to him exclusively and he will respond to it positively, providing it is to his advantage. If that were not true, T. S. Eliot would never have bothered writing the poem "The Naming of Cats" in *Old Possum's Book of Practical Cats*, from which the Broadway musical *Cats* is derived.

If you have not yet named your cat, it is best to use a short, sweet name that consists of just a couple of syllables, so it can be identified more easily. If you call your cat something like Newton's Law of Motion, chances are you're going to draw a blank when you call him. Not even Newton would respond to that. It is also important to understand that a cat will only respond to his name if a bond has been established between you. A bond involves a relationship of love and affection. Without it, nothing will work.

One begins training a cat by teaching him his name. A cat learns his name by hearing it repeatedly and associating the name with something pleasant. One must never use the cat's name in vain, for punishment or for scolding. The cat's name is useful when you want him to come to you. If the association is negative, no cat, dog, or child (or anyone else for that matter) will come running to your call. When teaching the cat his name, dole out a food reward every time it's said and praise him lavishly. Have faith. This really works.

COME WHEN CALLED

Once the cat learns his name, he is practically trained to come when called. Place him at one end of your home and yourself at the other end. Call him by name and offer him a treat and some affectionate praise if he comes to you. An effective reinforcement reward is a yeast tablet. Most cats adore them, and they are quite healthy when given in moderation. One or two at a time is the reward to give during any training session. A high-quality catnip also makes a good training reward, but should not be given until after the session. Some cats take a while to recover from the stimulating effect; others simply fall asleep.

HOUSE TRAINING

Most cats and kittens arrive in their new homes as trained ladies and gentlemen who have been taught toilet manners by their mothers. However, there are those who have not had enough time with mama cat to know what it's all about. Cats can be easily house trained and expected to remain clean and well trained. It is what they prefer. To house train a cat simply place him in his cat box (refer to Chapter Two, "A Kitten in Your Life"), move his front paws in the filler, and encourage him to scratch it. Nature will take over. In a matter of minutes your cat will use the box as his toilet and you'll be in business.

Obviously, you will need a cat box. They are available in pet supply stores, hardware stores, and in some food markets. The most common filler for the box is granulated clay, which is commercially manufactured and sold in all supermarkets. It is generically referred to as cat litter.

The newest cat-box filler on the market is unscented granules with the consistency of fine sand and captures liquid waste before it can reach the bottom of the box or saturate the litter, turning it into easy-to-remove balls. Since odor-causing waste is eliminated, the box remains fresh and clean. One simply adds more litter as it is needed.

This product can be important for cat-box training because cats will not use a dirty toilet. One of the reasons for housebreaking problems is that cat boxes are not easy to keep clean and free of odors. Some cats do not like the feel of conventional litter, so they just won't use it. But many cats love the sandy feel of this newer type, making it the perfect solution for house training or for cats with litter-box problems.

"NO!"

"No" is more of a demand than a command. It is a negatively learned lesson, but perhaps the most valuable one in the repertoire. Walking on your supper, climbing the curtains, using your leg or your couch for a scratch post—all call for a firmly taught respect for the command "NO!"

Whenever your cat transgresses, lift him by the scruff of the neck as his mother would do, support is back legs with your palm, shake him firmly, and say, "No, No, No" in a firm tone of voice. If the cat was scratching you or the furniture, immediately take him to his scratch post (refer to Chapter Two, "A Kitten in Your Life") and work his front paws on it in a teaching fashion. Then reward him with a treat and some praise. When trying to redirect misbehavior, show the cat what he is supposed to do and then reward him and praise him. Corrections are not enough.

Eventually, saying "No" in a firm voice will suffice without the shaking. Consistency is very important. Once you begin disciplining with the word "No," use that word exclusively for that purpose and no other. In that way, the word becomes an effective training tool. You can extend your omnipotence with the use of a water pistol or a strong squirt bottle. If you are across the room and the cat decides to scratch the corner of the carpet or the front of the sofa, you can stop him and teach him at the same time. Give him a squirt of the water (not in the eyes) and say, "No, no, no" in a loud, firm tone of voice.

The independent air of most cats is quite justified because of their ability to resort to predatory skills if forced to return to the wild state. However, house cats need humans to feed them, clean their litter boxes, let them in and out, supply the catnip, and shield them from galloping dogs and clutchy children. It is within these domestic needs that cat training becomes possible.

CHAPTER SIX

A Good-Looking Cat

Grooming your cat is a matter of health and happiness, yours as well as hers. A well-groomed pet is more than a thing of beauty, she is a shining example of loving care. Grooming immeasurably improves the quality of the animal's health and will add years to your cat's life.

Anyone would expect a cat named Algernon, Havisham, or Melissa to be quite prim and proper—svelte or fluffy, too. But even roughnecks like Mulligan, Mazy, or Spike need to be kept in line with a spit and polish attitude from the caring owner. Good grooming, after all, means good health. An ungroomed cat will shed fur in your omelet and smudge paw prints on your fine linens and upholstery. Because owners of companion cats have no need for show grooming techniques as a rule and because the subject can fill a book of its own, only those grooming needs that keep a furry friend healthy and reasonably pleasing aesthetically are offered here.

Without a doubt, the most desirable of all options is an occasional visit to a professional groomer. These are trained and skilled animal technicians who have a great deal to offer the busy pet owner. For people out of the house all day and tired at night, the professional groomer is a blessing. For those who have the time, energy, and inclination to learn how to keep their cats healthy, clean, and good-looking, this chapter will help you to do it.

Grooming does more than keep your cat looking good, though. When you groom your cat properly, you are actually practicing preventive medicine. When you or a professional grooms your cat, you are also examining your pet's body. In that way you can detect potential problems that can seriously affect your cat's health. In the course of grooming you can examine your cat from nose to tail and look for parasites, lumps under the skin, infections, rashes, dental problems, and even minor injuries. Combing and brushing down to the skin enable this kind of in-depth, external examination, which even a veterinarian cannot give.

Cat grooming primarily refers to giving your cat a bath, cleaning his ears and eyes, clipping his nails, and cleaning his teeth. It is true, however, that some long-haired cats must have their coats trimmed a bit, and that usually requires the services of a professional groomer.

YOUR CAT'S SKIN AND COAT

The Skin

Before you can effectively keep your cat groomed, you will need a working knowledge of your cat's skin and coat. Obviously, the skin is the external covering of your cat's body and holds everything together that is beneath it. It is a waterproof shield that prevents most diseases from entering the body and controls the body's temperature as well.

The skin is the largest organ in all mammals and is comprised of the *epidermis,* which is the outer layer; the *dermis,* which is the underlying support structure directly beneath the *epidermis;* and the *subcutis,* which is found beneath the *dermis* and is made of fibers that cover the fatty tissue beneath the skin.

The Hair

A single hair is a lengthy, delicate, threadlike structure made of an inert substance called *keratin.* Its composition includes a hollow, tubular shaft and a root. The root is held in a *follicle* or sac which is attached beneath the surface of the skin past the dermis and the subcutaneous layer. Attached to the hair follicles are the *arrector pili muscles*, which originate in the *dermis*. When they contract, they cause the hair to stand erect, which happens when cats are emotionally stressed or in a fighting stance.

Also attached to the bulb-shaped hair follicle are *sebaceous glands*, which secrete *sebum,* a thick fluid that travels up each hair shaft, providing a protective coating and giving the hair a lustrous appearance. The sebum not only covers the outer hair surface but seeps out onto the skin itself, keeping it soft and pliable. When a cat's hair coat becomes dull and dry, it is often due to malfunctioning sebaceous glands, which may be caused by sickness, poor diet, or the presence of parasites in or on the body. In many such instances, daily brushing and combing stimulates the glands into secreting their beneficial fluids, restoring their protective influence.

SHEDDING

Shedding fur is simply dead hair, which clings to carpeting, upholstery fabric, and clothing. Hair that has shed from your cat dulls the most vivid colors and acts as a dragnet for dirt and dust. Flying fur and dander make some people cough and sneeze, while others become teary-eyed and itchy-skinned. Because cats are members of the family, we accept shedding with a resigned grin. Understanding why and how the shedding process works might help us live with it. There are a few ways to rid yourself of the problem with some cats and reduce it to manageable proportions with others.

The process of casting off one layer of hair and replacing it with another is more accurately termed *molting*. To molt is to replace hair, skin, horns, feathers, or scales after shedding the older covering. It is common throughout the animal kingdom. With hair-covered animals such as cats, nature's purpose is to replace the heavy winter coat with a lighter summer one. As the weather becomes colder, the reverse takes place. It is all a matter of insulation.

Shedding the winter coat begins in the spring, and under normal conditions takes approximately three weeks. Shedding the summer coat and replacing it with the heavier winter *pelage* occurs in autumn, preparing the animal for cold weather. Some breeds of cat molt just once a year, throughout a long cycle that achieves the same effect. It is commonly accepted that molting is influenced by the length of time spent outdoors exposed to the natural sequences of light and darkness. Shedding and regrowth begin in spring as the days get longer (more time spent in daylight) and again in late summer as the days shorten (less time spent in daylight).

Feline coats are affected by the pituitary gland, which is influenced by the ratio of light to darkness. This influence may be exerted chemically, photoelectrically, or mechanically and is informally referred to as a body clock. Although not yet established by medical research, it is suspected that abnormal shedding cycles may be caused by a cat's indoor life, which involves irregular exposure to light and darkness. Pets exposed to prolonged periods under their owners' electric lights may have extended molting cycles and shed continuously.

Females often shed more than males because of the activity of the pituitary gland during the estrus cycles (*heat* or periods of sexual receptivity). They have been known to shed almost their entire coats shortly after bearing a litter of kittens. Shedding cycles diminish in intensity and frequency as the female ages and goes into estrus less frequently. This may not be true, however, if an aging female spends long periods of time under artificial lights.

Shedding may also be the result of physiological or emotional stress or disease. Constant or intense shedding may indicate a sick animal. Watch for signs such as itching, slackened appetite, dull coat, or bald patches. If they appear, call your veterinarian. Other factors that influence shedding are internal or external parasites; poor or imbalanced diets; intense indoor heating; and even friction from tight-fitting collars.

The question always arises, which breed of cat sheds more or less than others. Few experts will disagree that all felines shed at least once a year and that many cats shed continuously throughout the year. One breed of cat, a real eye-catcher, is said not to shed at all—the Rex. Inasmuch as all mammals shed hair, it is perhaps more accurate to say that the Rex sheds less than other cats. Another breed that sheds little or not at all is the very rare Sphynx, which is practically hairless. It has no coat, only warm skin with small amounts of hair on the bridge of the nose, behind the ears, on the feet, and on the upper part of the tail. Its coat pattern is skin pigmentation rather than hair. Shedding is a fact of life, however, for just about all cats, no matter which breed.

Nothing will prevent your cat from shedding his old coat. However, there are several ways to reduce the impact. Keep your cat in good health with regular exercise, frequent veterinary checkups, examinations for parasites, and a well-balanced diet (available in premium commercial pet foods). Give him an occasional teaspoon of cooked animal fat or a commercial food supplement meant for coat maintenance. Daily brushing and combing plus an occasional bath do the most to rid the animal of dead hair and loose dander. It is also helpful to apply a commercial coat conditioner to relieve dry skin, dull coat, and shedding hair.

How to Avoid the Problem of Shedding

All cats rotate their coats twice a year. They regrow one coat as they lose the old one, at the same time. Unfortunately, the process seems to continue all year long because all the "blown" or dead hair does not fall out right away. There is always falling hair in the house whether you live with an American Shorthair or a Persian. Shedding can be avoided, if not totally eliminated, by giving your cat a hot-to-warm-water bath and a thorough comb-out. Use a cream rinse for long-coated cats or cats with a dense undercoat. After the bath, towel the excess water off the cat's body. Next, use a warm-air blow dryer for as long as it takes to dry the coat. Use the Low setting and move the blow dryer back and forth along the cat's coat, but do not get it too close. As you blow-dry, comb out the coat vigorously. The comb must penetrate down to the skin on all parts of the body. The warm air will force out onto your comb most of the dead hair, the dying hair, and the loose hair. The hair that you remove with this technique is the hair that would have been shed in your house over a long period of time. Do this twice a year, just as the coat is about to rotate.

HOW TO GROOM YOUR CAT FOR GOOD LOOKS AND GOOD HEALTH

Trimming Your Cat's Nails

It is essential to trim your cat's nails frequently for several reasons. First, it helps your pet get rid of the outer nail sheath and allows the incoming nails to emerge without discomfort. Second, it avoids destructive behavior toward your furniture because you have helped the cat remove the outer, dead nail, thus removing his need to scratch (for a while, anyway). Third, humans are less likely to be seriously injured once the cat's claws are blunted through trimming.

Always trim your cat's nails before grooming sessions and baths.

Feline claws are unique because they are retractable and do not show in their usual, retracted position. When cats walk, only the very tips occasionally come in contact with the ground. The claws are formidable weapons and are extended when the cat prepares to fight, run, or climb. The claws are also unsheathed when the animal is frightened or panicked. Unsheathed claws are necessary for catching prey animals. Tree climbing, jumping, escape maneuvers, playing, fighting, mating, and many other activities also involve the retractabile claws.

When a cat scratches on a scratch post or on your furniture, she is obeying an important impulse to remove the outer layer of the tissue and make room for the continuously growing nail underneath. You can avoid much of the damage to yourself and your possessions by keeping the nails trimmed. They should be trimmed at least once a week and before every bath.

You will need a tool that is designed to trim your cat's nails with ease. Feline nail trimmers come in three types. There is the *scissor type*, which is small with blunt ends instead of points. The blades form a circular hole in which you place the claw and then snip. There is the *safety nail trimmer*, which resembles a pair of pliers with a spring between the handles. It, too, functions as a scissors with a circular hole in the blades, but it has a safety stop to limit the length of the nail cut. And there is the *guillotine trimmer*, a cross between a pair of pliers and a cigar cutter. The nail is placed in the hole at the end of the tool and the handles are squeezed together, causing a sharp blade to slide across, slicing off the exposed bit of nail.

Once you have the proper tool, you are ready to clip your cat's nails. The trick to trimming is to put gentle pressure on the nails so that they extend out of the skin covering. Place the cat's paw on your open palm. Select the nail that needs trimming and rest your thumb against the corresponding toe. The nail will appear. If the nails are a quarter inch past the pink area, they should be clipped. Most cat nails are white or buff-colored at the tips and pink as they get closer to the base. The pink area is called the *quick;* it indicates where the nerve endings are located and where the blood vessels begin. You must never clip the nails at the quick. If you do, you will cause pain and slight bleeding. In dark-haired cats, some or all of the nails may be black or darker than usual. This will make it difficult to avoid the quick. If you trim the nail just at the curve, you will avoid any problems.

Once the nails have been clipped with the cutting tool, it is a good idea to smooth down the sharp edges as you would when cutting your own nails, with an emery board and nail buffer. Some cat owners use the emery board exclusively as a way of keeping the nails in trim. It does work, even though it is more time-consuming.

Bathing Your Cat

Few cats enjoy baths. Even fewer cat owners enjoy giving them. Nothing makes a cat appear more miserable than standing in a bathtub all soaped up and scrawny-looking. Although we may think of baths as part of the glamour/grooming process designed for show cats, they have more to do with cleanliness and keeping your cat healthy.

The most frequently asked bath question is How often is it necessary? The next most asked question: Are baths harmful? Opinion differs on both questions, from professional groomers, veterinarians, breeders, and experienced cat owners. It is safe to say that a bath is necessary when the cat smells bad, is absolutely filthy, has gotten into something greasy or foul, or when a good appearance is desired for some special occasion. Some professionals maintain that once a month is good, while others say that once a year or even once a lifetime is better. How often to bathe a cat depends on the type of coat your cat has, its color and texture, the cat's living conditions, how often you brush the cat, and how well you keep him clean. Some professional groomers advise you to bathe your cat every couple of months. Allow common sense to guide you. If you brush and comb your cat properly on a daily basis and remove dead hair before it can mat, you will not have to bathe the cat frequently. As suggested before, bathe a cat twice a year if you have a shedding problem. (See "Shedding" earlier in this chapter.)

If your cat is dirty or smells bad give him a bath. That is probably the best policy. If you select a high quality shampoo that is the correct one for your cat you can bathe your pet as frequently as you want without having him suffer any ill effects.

Too many baths can remove the oils produced by the sebaceous glands, thus drying out your cat's skin and coat. A dry coat has lost its waterproofing effect in addition to looking bad. This can create a dry skin condition that causes itching, and minor irritation or infection from scratching. Some cats are bathed three times or less throughout their lives, while others are bathed more than once a month. It is a personal choice based on the individual cat's requirements and your use of the right shampoos, rinses, and conditioners. Cats with allergies or infections will need to be bathed as directed by a veterinarian, and most country cats require a flea and tick dip during the summer.

How old should a cat be before you bathe her? Opinion seems to vary from expert to expert. Consider the facts. Veterinarians believe that all kittens are vulnerable to upper respiratory illnesses if they are exposed to drafts or chills. Standing in a tub, soaked to the skin, can make any cat sick if the room temperature is not warm enough or if there is a draft. For this reason some experts believe a kitten should not be bathed for the first ten months of its life. Others feel six months is adequate for safety's sake, while others say one-day-old is a good time to begin baths if the conditions are correct.

The alternatives to frequent bathing are easy and highly effective. First, you can remove superficial dirt from a cat with a damp washcloth. Gummy substances can be removed with witch hazel on a dampened cloth. Then there are dozens of commercially prepared ''dry shampoos'' that work well with a good brushing. For light-colored, longhaired cats you can sprinkle cornstarch or Fullers Earth throughout the fur by parting the coat in many places. Shake the powder onto all parts of the body except the head. After a heavy application, confine the cat for fifteen minutes to allow the powder to absorb the excess body oil and dirt, then use a clean, soft brush to remove the powder and the dirt at the same time. A simple, thorough brushing every day will do more to keep a cat clean than all the baths she'll ever get.

If your white Persian looks like stale Wonder Bread or your shorthaired tabby resembles the inside of a vacuum cleaner bag, it's time for a dip, a scrub, and a rinse. The cat will agree, but only *after* the bath. She may not cooperate. That's why it will probably take two of you to accomplish a bath, especially if it is a first-time experience.

What you'll need to bathe your cat

Sink or small plastic tub
Small window screen

Bath mat
Cat shampoo
Plastic cup
Portable spray hose (optional)
Detangling liquid (for cats with matted fur)
Mineral oil
Absorbent cotton
Stainless steel cat comb (half fine–half medium is recommended)
Natural-bristle brush (some prefer a rubber curry brush for shorthaired cats)
Electric hair dryer (type used by humans)
Three or four large towels
Cat carrier (for confinement during the drying process)

You will need a commercially manufactured, pH-balanced shampoo that says on the label that it was formulated for cats. By paying attention to the pH factor, you will help keep your cat's skin and coat in the best condition possible. Stay away from shampoos and other products that were formulated for humans, dogs, or other creatures. Always use a *cat* shampoo.

The pH factor has to do with the acidity or alkalinity of the product, which is measured on a pH scale running from 0 to 14, with 7 being neutral. 0 to 7 is acid; 7 to 14 is alkaline. Human hair requires "non-alkaline" or "acid balanced" shampoos (0–7 pH). Cats require a slightly more alkaline-based shampoo for their skin and hair (6.2–8.6 pH). That is why human shampoos, even those made for babies, are not the best ones to use for your cat. Among the vast array of cat shampoos there are mild, tearless shampoos for kittens and cats with sensitive skin, shampoos formulated for various coat colors, shampoos for adding body or texture to the coat, medicated shampoos for use on cats with various skin disorders, coal tar shampoos for cats with seborrhea, and flea and tick shampoos.

Other bath products worth using are cream rinses and conditioners. These help control shedding coats, repair damaged hairs, add luster to the surface of the hair, soften the coat, and help prevent tangling, making the coat easier to brush. There are also lotions, hair moisturizers, and super conditioners worth trying; their labels are self-explanatory.

After-bath coat conditioners and coat dressings help create a better appearance while making the hair easier to brush. A coat conditioner has oil among its other ingredients. A dressing has no oil. All of these products add greatly to the strength of the hair while conditioning it.

Preparation. Close all windows and doors so the cat cannot leave the room if he should escape your grip. Clip the cat's nails before doing anything, to lessen the possibility of serious injury.

Always brush and comb your cat out just before a bath. Make sure that all the loose hair is out of the coat before it becomes wet with bathwater. If you do not brush out your cat's coat before the bath, it will be difficult to get rid of the dead hair afterward, and the coat will be hard to dry out because it will knot up and get lumpy. This is especially important if your cat has long hair or is shedding.

If the cat's coat has mats or tangles in it, they should be removed before the bath is given. First, use a fine-wire *slicker brush* to break up the mats into smaller clumps. Next, use a fine-tooth comb with a commercial detangling liquid to break the mats apart completely.

The kitchen or bathroom sink is the ideal tub for a cat bath because of its height. Set up the small window screen inside the sink so that it slants against one edge. The cat will be placed on it during the bath so that he can keep his balance by digging into the mesh with his nails. A folded towel or a rubber mat placed on the bottom of the sink along with the screen is best.

Place a few drops of mineral oil in your cat's eyes to prevent soap or shampoo burns. You may also loosely stuff a wad of absorbent cotton in each ear canal to prevent water from running in.

Now the bath. Fill the sink one-third full with tepid water and add a small quantity of cat shampoo. Adding shampoo to the water helps to wet down the cat more easily by getting directly to the skin. Cat hair tends to resist moisture. Place the cat in the sink and allow her to stand on the screen for traction. One person should hold her while the other works with the shampoo and water. Once the cat is in the sink, take a plastic cup and pour the slightly soapy water over her. If there are no fleas to deal with, do not wet the head until last, because it's the most frightening part for the cat. However, wet the head first if the animal is infested with any form of parasite. When the body becomes wet, the fleas will scurry to the head area, where it becomes difficult to get them out.

Talk to Tabby in a quiet, reassuring tone of voice as you work. With any luck, the cat will be calmed by the time you're ready for the head. With the hair wet, apply the cat shampoo of your choice, rubbing it in with your fingertips. Get all the way down to the skin and clean the body with a massaging action much as you would shampoo your own head.

Work up a good lather and get it deep into the coat and onto the skin. Massage the shampoo into the shoulders, down the back and the legs, between the toes, up and on the underbody and, finally, the tail. Gently scrub the head and the ears, being careful around the eyes, then under the chin and down the neck into the front bib. When a cat stands in bathwater with a little shampoo added to it the paws are automatically softening and getting cleaned, especially between the toes. If the paws are sore or afflicted with an irritation or a fungus, then add a medicated cat shampoo to the bathwater.

You are now ready to rinse the shampoo off of the body. Use the hand spray or portable spray hose but do not use it on the cat's head or face. Start at the head and go down the back to the sides of the body, and then the legs, so all the soapy, dirty water runs off the cat and does not simply pour onto another part of his body.

If the cat is very dirty a second shampoo is desirable and should be given immediately, but do not shampoo twice unless it is absolutely necessary. Never keep a cat in water longer than you have to.

A professional groomer's trick for making combing and

brushing easier after a bath is to use a cream rinse during the final stages. Simply follow the manufacturer's instructions on the label. Empty out any water remaining in the sink and refill it with clear, tepid water. Rinse the cat once more until you see clear water coming of her body. Take a large towel and blot-dry the body, getting rid of the excess moisture. Using a second towel, remove the cat from the sink and towel-dry her instantly so that she does not get chilled. With your fingers and the towel you may gently squeeze the water out of the coat. Try not to create tangles during any part of the drying process. Continue to towel-dry until the cat is no longer dripping wet.

It is now time to use the electric hair dryer. Use it with the blower on but with the heat set on Low. For shorthaired cats brush with a soft, natural-bristle brush or rubber brush as you work with the dryer. The drying motion requires short, quick strokes with the brush and the dryer. For long-haired cats do not let the warm air flow on the coat without using a brush or comb. Apply a fluff-dry technique, that is, brush or comb the fur with long, flowing strokes in upward motions. This has the effect of lifting the hair and allowing the underside of the hairs to benefit from the heat. It is also what creates a fluffy coat.

Do not allow the cat to roam around while she is still damp. This may chill her and will only get her dirty all over again. Line the bottom of your cat carrier with a clean towel and place your pet inside until she is completely dry. Keep her warm and free from drafts. Remember, longhaired cats need more drying time than shorthaired cats.

It is now time to give Balthazar a treat of some kind for putting up with a disagreeable experience. You may now commence to comb and brush her, spray a coat conditioner on her, tie a ribbon around her neck, and let her watch the birds from your living-room window.

Daily Brushing and Combing

The hair coat creates the outer beauty of all cats, and by brushing and combing it on a regular basis you can keep it clean and good-looking. A cat that is brushed regularly and correctly will not need frequent bathing. This can be important for some cats whose coats tend to become dry from baths. For many cat owners grooming is a matter of good looks, but one must consider grooming from a health point of view first and as a beauty treatment second. At the very least, dirt on a cat's body can cause a variety of skin ailments that can become serious. Bear in mind that whatever is in or on a cat's body will eventually get into the human living areas where she spends many hours each day and night. Some cats lick themselves and swallow all manner of debris this way. They may swallow anything from parasites to broken glass. For these reasons a cat should be brushed every day, and combed out if it is appropriate for your cat's coat. *Daily brushing removes dead hair, and daily combing removes or prevents minor mats and tangles (preventing them from developing into serious problems).* Combing also smooths out the coat in a pleasing way. The skin beneath the fur should be inspected when the cat is being groomed and checked for lumps, cuts, or lesions.

Groomers, breeders, and exhibitors who show their cats refer to a dull, lifeless, shedding coat as "blown." A "blown coat," however, is easily dealt with by getting rid of the loose and dead hair with a slicker brush or steel comb. Daily maintenance of a "blown coat" is important in order to prevent difficult and painful mats and tangles from developing.

When you brush and comb your cat frequently, you remove dirt, dust, and dead hair. You also help spread the secreted oils from the sebaceous glands that are so beneficial for the hair and skin. Daily brushing and combing also massages the skin and stimulates new hair growth. And, finally, regular brushing and combing keeps the skin free from external parasites.

GROOMING TOOLS

Brushes

Bristle brush. This is the one grooming tool needed by everyone for the care of long-, medium-, and short-coated cats.

A natural bristle brush is made of bristles that are graduated in length so they can penetrate the coat more efficiently. All bristle brushes come in a variety of sizes and shapes, with soft, medium, or stiff bristles. The one you select should be based on your cat's size, coat length, and coat texture. Common sense will guide you.

The best bristle brushes have all-natural bristles that are set directly into a wooden backing rather than a rubber one. Soft, natural bristles are best because they reduce friction and avoid discomfort for the cat and the static electricity that helps create mats and tangles. A combination natural and nylon bristle brush is a decent compromise if economy is an important consideration. Nylon bristle brushes are not recommended for cats because of their tendency to irritate their delicate skin.

Fine-wire slicker brush. Rectangular in shape, these have wooden handles. Slicker brushes are characterized by short, bent-wire teeth placed closely together, resembling the metal fins inside an air conditioner. Although they are available in many sizes, a small to medium size is best to use for cats. Their purpose is to untangle mats and remove dead hair from cats with long coats, such as Persians and Maine Coon Cats. Be certain you purchase a *fine-wire* slicker brush meant for cats and delicate dogs.

Hard rubber brush. Made of one molded piece of rubber that includes the teeth, this brush is for grooming and polishing short-coated and smooth-coated cats. The rubber brush can also be used for shampooing and massaging without scratching or irritating the sensitive skin of cats. It is of little or no use in grooming long- or medium-coated cats.

Soft-bristle toothbrush. This is especially useful for longhair cats. It is used to scrub the facial area if there is eye stain.

Soft brush. A separate, soft brush with a handle is necessary for maintaining a white or light-colored long-haired coat. This brush is used exclusively for brushing in and then brushing out cornstarch, Fuller's Earth, or other powder when dry cleaning the coat.

Chamois cloth. Many coats are made more beautiful by polishing them after they are brushed. Some coats are too fine for brushing, and a wipe with a chamois adds the finishing touch. A silk scarf or piece of velvet will also provide the necessary luster when rubbed into the coat.

Combs

There is a wide variety of combs to choose from. One should buy the best quality for ease of handling, durability, and comfort of the cat. Cat combs made of stainless steel or chrome-plated brass are best. There are some high-quality aluminum combs available, but be certain the points of the teeth are smooth and rounded, not harsh or sharp. It is desirable to match the length and spacing of the teeth to the character-istics of your cat's coat. Long coats require a comb with longer teeth than short, silky coats.

Half-medium, half-fine comb. This is the most useful comb to own because it can be used for most breeds and coat types. The fine teeth are for soft or silky hair; the medium teeth are for coats of average texture. Both medium and fine teeth are often used on different sections of the same cat's coat. Half-medium, half-fine combs are made in various sizes to accommodate almost any type of coat, of just about any size cat. The shape and design of the half-medium, half-fine comb resembles a typical comb found in anyone's bathroom. The length of the teeth on the comb you buy should depend on the length of your cat's coat.

Medium Belgium comb with a handle. This can be very useful for grooming long-haired cats. The handle makes lifting the coat, layer by layer, easier to accomplish. The ends of the teeth should be rounded so they do not cause painful scratches or serious skin irritations.

Fine-tooth comb with a handle. This comb can be used for both short- and long-haired cats. It is especially useful for combing out the area around the head of long-haired cats.

HOW TO BRUSH AND COMB YOUR CAT

Short-Coat

A short-coated cat with smooth hair does not require a great deal of grooming. Remember, the object of brushing is to remove dead and loose hair as often as you can. A short-coated cat with coarse hair will probably have an abundance of dead hair to remove and will require more time.

It is *not* a good idea to brush the coat when it is dry. You are advised to moisten the coat before starting out the daily brushing and combing routine. A spritz of coat conditioner or dressing is ideal, but as an alternative you may run a bit of water through the coat with your fingers as though giving a massage. Water is better than nothing at all and is fairly effective. Once the coat is *slightly* moistened use a quality bristle brush or a hard rubber brush. All kittens require a soft-bristle brush.

Work the brush through the coat with long, gentle strokes, taking as much dead and loose hair with you as possible. Be sure to stroke the entire body from shoulder to toes, from nose to tail. Work the brush gently but with the necessary pressure to move the hair in whichever direction you're going. Swing your hand, wrist, and entire arm in whatever direction you're brushing with a long, stroking movement. Each brush stroke should be part of a steady, rhythmical movement that is comfortable for you and the cat. If you do this with a steady, sweeping motion, you can brush your cat without tiring for as long as it takes to do a thorough job.

Some short coats consist of a single coat, and others are double. The single coat is sleek and shiny and with a delicate texture. It lies flat against the skin. The double coat has long hairs on the top that display the color and pattern and a short, fluffy, dense coat on the belly. Double-coated cats tend to shed more. Daily brushing, massaging, and combing are important.

After brushing, run a comb through the coat, starting at the head and working to the tail, in the natural direction of the growth. Do not neglect the stomach, legs, tail, and head. Afterward you may use a coat conditioner or dressing. Finish the session by polishing the coat with a chamois cloth. All short-coated cats should look smooth and shiny. All double-coated cats should look soft and luxurious.

Long-Coat

Moisten the coat before starting out the daily combing and brushing routine. Do not groom a dry coat. A spritz of coat conditioner or dressing is ideal, but as an alternative you may run a bit of water through the coat with your fingers as though giving a massage. Massage the skin gently with your fingers in order to loosen dead hairs.

Long-haired coats should generally be combed first and then brushed. The main point to combing *any* coat type is to remove mats and tangles and smooth out the coat. Combing also helps remove dirt and dead hair. All long hair must be combed out thoroughly to remove and prevent mats and tangles. A professional groomer's trick for making this task easier is to use a cream rinse during the final stages of a bath.

Starting with the trunk, comb the longest hair with the medium-tooth portion of the comb. Work upward and outward as you stroke the back, sides, and behind the legs. Get the teeth deep into the hair and close to the skin and carefully lift upward as you comb the fur out. Do not forget to comb the flanks, belly, and entire leg areas. Take the end of the tail in your fingers and shake it carefully. Use the medium portion of the comb for the tail and groom with the lay of the fur.

The fine-tooth comb is to be used on the forehead and around the ears in an upward and forward direction; cheek hair should be guided forward and outward. Comb the feet and the legs with the fine-tooth portion of the combination comb. Stroke protruding leg hair in an upward direction. Comb the long tufts of fur between the toes upward with the fine-tooth comb.

As a final step, use your soft, natural-bristle brush to gently stroke with the lay of the fur, using short movements, from the shoulder to the haunch to the tail. The brush should catch any remaining dead hair while applying the finishing touches.

Daily combing and brushing will help prevent tangles, knots, and mats in the fur of the long-haired cat. The amount of matting depends on the texture and length of the fur. Coarse hair, for example, will not mat as readily as fine hair. There are several fine detangling liquids available, to be used in conjunction with a fine-tooth comb or other detangling tool, that make mat removal much easier.

Here is some advice about how to stroke the brush. Work the brush gently but with the necessary pressure to move the hair in whichever direction you're going. Swing your hand, wrist, and entire arm in whatever direction you're brushing with a long, stroking movement. Each brush stroke should be part of a steady, rhythmical movement that is comfortable for you and the cat. If you do this with a steady, sweeping motion, you can brush your cat without tiring for as long as it takes to do a thorough job.

TIPS ON COAT CARE

To remove eye stains (spots on the fur caused by tearing), clip the hair under the eyes. Then wash the hair with a no-tear shampoo and brush it out with a soft-bristle toothbrush. You can cover remaining stains with a siliconized chalk pencil designed for this purpose.

To remove chewing gum stuck in the coat, rub it with peanut butter and remove it after several minutes. Then comb out the residue. An optional method is to rub the gum with an ice cube. When it becomes brittle, break it apart and simply pull the pieces out.

When tar or viscous oil sticks to the coat or paws, soak the troubled area in warm water, then drench it with mineral oil. Repeat this until the tar loosens and yields to vigorous wiping.

Skunk odor or other such horrors can be gotten rid of by rubbing tomato juice or vanilla extract into the coat. Leave it on for one or two hours. Give the cat a thorough shampoo and rinse. It may be necessary to repeat this procedure.

CARE OF THE EARS

Your cat's ears make her vulnerable to various medical conditions that can be irritating, painful, and even dangerous. Medically, one must watch for parasitic ear mites, which are microscopic parasites that resemble insects when examined under a microscope but are actually members of the spider family. They are barely visible. Head shaking, ear scratching, restless behavior, and the presence of brown, waxy material in the ear canal are the signs. Consult a veterinarian for treating this condition. It is a good idea to look inside your cat's ears at least once a month.

When checking your cat's ears, clean out wax deposits with a cloth wrapped around your finger or with a cotton swab dipped in baby oil or peroxide. (There are commercial products available for this purpose.) *Do not penetrate too deeply into the canal lest you cause an injury to the inner skin or delicate parts of the ear.* After cleansing the inner portion of the ear, use an antiseptic powder inside to help prevent infection.

Cats should have their ears routinely cleaned. If your cat does not accept ear cleaning very well, have someone help you. Wrap the cat's body in a towel so that all four paws are restrained, and have your assistant hold her firmly. Only the head should extend out of the towel. Proceed with the ear cleaning. If there is a great accumulation of ear wax, do not attempt to clean it out yourself unless you are very experienced.

CARE OF THE EYES

Some cat are mores susceptible to eye injury or irritations than others. They need extra eye care. Look for specks of dirt or debris that may get into the eyeball and cause discomfort. If you cannot remove them, see a veterinarian.

Occasionally cats have trouble with eyelashes that grow inward, onto the eye. To prevent this, the eyelashes may require a bit of careful wiping. Untrimmed facial hair may also rub into the eyeball, causing irritation, infection, and, in some extreme cases, ulceration. Consult a professional groomer or a veterinarian.

Some cats' eyes tear all the time. If that is not normal for your cat, a discharge from her eyes is usually a sign of irritation, infection, or some ailment in the body. See a veterinarian if the condition does not clear up in a day or two. The *haw* or third eyelid closes laterally in some types of eye problems and makes the eye appear to be covered with a translucent film. Medicated eye solution for cats or boric acid solution can be dropped or wiped into the eyes, but a visit to the veterinarian is the best thing.

If your cat suddenly develops a teary-eyed condition from pollution in the air, pollen, or grass seed, wipe the eyes with a clean, soft cloth dipped in a weak solution of warm water and boric acid. Apply the cloth to the corners of the eyes and wipe outward, away from the eye.

Cats with light-colored coats are often stained with a brownish discoloration on the facial hair around the eyes. This is caused by continual tearing. Ask a veterinarian if there is any medical reason for the tearing. From a grooming point of view daily care is the main solution to the problem. Comb the hair under the eyes with a fine tooth comb to clean away solid matter. Next, every day use a liquid solution that is formulated to soothe the eyes of cats. Apply a few drops onto the stained hairy areas beneath the eyes, as well as placing some in the eyes. Professional groomers often elect to trim away some of the unsightly hair and then color the remaining stains with a chalklike product to conceal it. In many cases, this is the best you can do.

If you are interested in total cat grooming, you are advised to consult a professional groomer or refer to a cat grooming manual. An alternative is to attend cat shows and watch the exhibitors and handlers in the benching area as they work on their beautiful show cats. Get acquainted with these people and don't be afraid to ask them questions. There is much to learn about this intriguing subject.

CHAPTER SEVEN

The Healthy Cat

The health needs of cats are much different from the needs of humans—or are they? A cat requires a clean environment to maintain a germ-free condition. So does a human. A cat must maintain some form of muscle tone so that fat does not interfere with the blood's transportation of oxygen and nutrients to the living cells. The same applies to a human. A cat is obsessed with a sense of personal hygiene through self-grooming or preening behavior, although no one understands why. With some qualifications, the same can be said for a human. Self-grooming and certain forms of social grooming are behavioral traits that every mammal shares one way or another. That would tend to give us a great deal in common with our favorite pet, the cat.

The stresses and strains of life as we live it have their bad effect on cats as they do on humans. Poor home life, eating the wrong food, eating too much, lack of exercise, little or no medical care, unnecessary stress all add up to a bad health picture. Pet owners should be as concerned about a cat's quality of life as about its longevity, a good prescription for living that applies to people as well as cats.

KEEPING YOUR CAT HAPPY

The first thing a healthy cat requires is a happy home life. It is not a difficult thing to achieve. Pet owners are unaware of the *little cruelties* they impose and are, themselves, as innocent as their four-legged companions.

Does love really mean never having to say you're sorry? You won't have to if you never hit your cat. Who could look at themselves in the mirror after bullying an innocent member of the family? It is probably a fact that most cat lovers are nonviolent and would never dream of abusing the animals they live with. And yet, great numbers of unconscious acts of cruelty are committed daily against pets by those who cherish them the most.

The little cruelties begin with misconceptions about cat behavior. Cats, despite their seeming independence, crave closeness and loving attention. But they are often left alone as kittens for five, eight, or twelve hours a day. Even though they have a childlike passion for play, they are sometimes ignored or abandoned, for an entire day in some cases. Kittens that are left alone for long periods of time may develop behavior problems such as poor housebreaking, aggressiveness, shyness, phobias, destructive chewing and scratching, and other unpleasant habits. Cats whose behavior becomes unbearable to humans often lose their homes and suffer an uncertain fate.

The most common wrong directed against cats is the way they are trained. Novice cat owners and those who should know better fail to understand the difference between training dogs and training cats. They use the one-size-fits-all approach. If you holler at or strike your cat, he is going to fear you forever and never give you the behavior you want. Cats are not programmed by nature to please you. Dogs are like that, not cats. Cats require a much different approach. Although cats respond well to discipline, it must not be harsh. Please read Chapter Five, "The Cat Train," for more information. After yelling or hitting the cat, the inexperienced owner then fails to understand why the family pet runs away when he or she goes to pet him.

The worst of it occurs over house soiling. If pet owners understood that *urine-marking* is the way a cat establishes his territory (the same for *fecal-marking*), they might be less upset and cope with it more intelligently. Here, the school of journalism is applied by hitting the cat with a rolled-up newspaper. There is no Pulitzer Prize given for this. This behavior is abusive and only worsens the problem.

House training a cat involves establishing the proper place for toileting, with the help of a cat box that has litter in it; keeping it clean on a daily basis; removing the scent of previous "mistakes," no matter how faint the odor by using a deodorizing product; and understanding that cats express their anxiety by marking territory. Please read Chapter Five, "The Cat Train" and the section on territory in Chapter Two, "A Kitten in Your Life," for more information. Things become much more pleasant once house soiling problems are solved.

Stress is an emotional and physical reaction to an upsetting external event. It can be caused by disease, injury, hunger, death of a family member, change of any kind, fear, and anxiety. Stress is often associated with the "fight or flight" response to danger. When a cat experiences stress, his body releases hormones that stimulate the adrenal glands. This raises the blood pressure, increases the heartbeat, rushes more oxygen to the muscles, and releases sugar into the bloodstream for quick energy. It can be an exhausting, unpleasant, and harmful experience. Putting a cat in a stressful situation is not only unkind, it is unhealthy. Some forms of travel, excessive exercise, punishment, unfriendly behavior, exposure to excessive heat or cold, strange animals, and fear-provoking situations produce stress, which results in an increased susceptibility to illness, behavioral problems, and depression. The little cruelties can be just as harmful as the big ones.

Get to Know the Unconscious Cruelties

- Isolation from the family and other humans
- Being left alone for long periods of time
- Harsh and abusive treatment
- No house training or discipline
- Improper discipline (punishments)

- Fear-inducing activities (exposure to threatening animals, loud noises, overbearing strangers, unsupervised children, etc.)
- Lack of attention or expressions of affection and approval
- Imbalanced diet, improper feeding schedule

Cat Chat

Everyone should talk to his or her cat, especially a new kitten. It makes perfect sense and does a lot of good. But we're usually too bashful about it. Very few cat owners want to be seen doing it. What will people think? Talking to your cat is a lot better than talking to yourself.

Most people are impressed with anyone who can communicate with animals. But wowing your friends is not an important reason for cat chat. The point is to make your new cat happy. If you want to succeed with your new kitten, you must help him become part of the family, and that involves developing a meaningful relationship. Which brings us to the idea of *bonding*.

Bonding. Kittens are influenced by the way you treat them, by your moods, and how you behave in front of them. They are also influenced by what you say to them and how you say it. If you want your kitten to grow into a good cat, there is one thing that must come before training or even housebreaking. You must establish a bond between you and your cat, which is simply a loving relationship. Try to get your cat to feel that he belongs, that he is a welcome part of the family. Talking to him helps accomplish this.

Bonding is a natural condition between parents and children, humans and pets. When you successfully create a bond with your kitten, everything else falls neatly into place. House training becomes easier, behavior problems are fewer and less intense, and your cat becomes a much more enjoyable pet.

House training. Who can argue with the fact that a housetrained cat behaves much better than one who isn't? But don't expect a kitten or even some adult cats to respond to your demands the minute they come to live with you. One of the myths of owning a cat is the idea that you should *never spoil your kitten*. That's wrong. Sure, you have to control your little cat to avoid trouble. But if you impose strict discipline and never let him get away with anything, you will seriously hinder him from becoming a happy cat. More important, you will never experience the joy of bonding with your kitten, and that is to miss the best part of cat ownership. It all starts with cat talk.

Speaking cat. Kittens are like babies. They love to be held and happily gibbered at. You'll never go wrong talking to your cat. The verbal connection creates a happy relationship that lasts for a lifetime, if you work it right. Out of this will come the cat's willingness to accept your gentle discipline. Talking to your cat is the easiest thing in the world. All you have to do is learn to speak cat.

Although a cat's grasp of the English language is quite limited, the sound of your voice communicates almost everything. It's exactly like talking to a newborn baby. Don't be afraid to make a fool out of yourself. The cat won't mind.

Kittens listen attentively to your voice and lap it up. Do not use a harsh, loud, angry tone with your kitten. When you speak with a soft tone of voice, you soothe and calm your new friend. If you use a high-pitched falsetto sound with enthusiasm, the kitten will become happily curious, energized, and will respond with pleasure, like a baby being tickled under the chin. Whether your voice is soothing or playful, it creates an emotional line between you and your cat that promotes love and trust.

This is especially important during the transition from your kitten's former life to his new life in your home. Most cats will slip instantly into a happy frame of mind and will easily adapt to their new home when you talk to them with fun and approval. "What a good cat you are!" It's all about love.

ALLERGIC TO YOUR CAT

When you bond with your cat, he expects you to hold him, pet him, and play with him. How is that possible if you discover that you are allergic to your cat? It is a difficult, almost impossible situation. Or is it?

When your cat jumps on your shoulder and licks your ear, you may find yourself laughing with uncontrollable, itchy tears. When you walk into the room where your cat is sleeping, you may begin a string of sneezes that wrack your body. Obviously, something is wrong. You may be allergic to your cat—even if you've never had a reaction to him before. There is a time interval between exposure to feline antigens and one's response to them. This is referred to as a period of sensitization. It is the usual progression of allergy development before symptoms appear. Only clinical testing by a medical doctor specializing in allergies can confirm your ailment. The standard wisdom from many allergists if you are allergic is to get rid of the animal quickly, heartlessly. However, that method of therapy is slowly changing.

What Is an Allergy?

An allergy is an abnormal reaction to a substance that is ordinarily harmless to most people. Substances that cause allergies are called *allergens* or *antigens*. They may be food or drugs swallowed daily; pollen, grass seed, house dust, or animal dander breathed in; poison ivy, cosmetics, grooming aids, or detergents touching the skin; or, chemicals injected into the body, such as some vaccines, medicines, or animal bites and stings. Statistics indicate that millions of people suffer from allergies in one form or another. And anyone can be allergic to anything.

Pet Allergies

The patient who complains to the doctor of chronic discomfort from a stuffed or running nose, tearing eyes, itchy skin, coughing and wheezing, shortness of breath, eczema or hives probably has an allergy. It is painfully serious news to learn it may be caused by a pet. Often, the patient is advised to "get rid of the offending animal." For some this is unthinkable. Not only are the feelings of the patient involved, but also humane

considerations. Finding another home for a cat is difficult and
almost impossible if the animal is not young.

Still, allergic sensitivity to animals is among the most
frequently seen allergies in the United States, according to the
Asthma and Allergy Foundation of America. Generally, the
allergen stems from a dog or cat, but guinea pigs, mice, gerbils,
birds, and especially horses may be the source. Unfortunately,
no one is allergic to a substance with the first contact. Two
years (more or less) is the most common period of sensitization, in which an allergen slowly leads to full-blown symptoms.
There are also special situations where the allergy stems from
a combination of allergens that individually would not cause an
allergic reaction in the patient. This is an important fact. It may
be possible to avoid removing a pet if it only causes a reaction
in combination with house dust or spores living on old books,
for example. Consult an allergist.

It is important to understand how pets create allergic
reactions. Any feathered or furry animal can cause allergy
discomforts in humans. The animals that people are most
allergic to are cats, dogs, and horses (in that order), and hair
length has little bearing on the matter. People do not suffer
greater allergy symptoms from a Persian cat than from an
American Shorthair, or from an Afghan Hound as opposed to
a Poodle. Neither are allergies influenced by the quantity of
shedding.

The allergic response to a pet is more likely to come from its
dander than its hair. Dander is the microscopic scales of dead
skin that flake into the environment. It is similar to human
dandruff but much smaller, almost like dust or powder, and it
is constantly shed from *all* cats and dogs. Other significant pet
allergens are saliva and urine containing certain proteins. Cats
cause greater allergic reactions because they deposit large
quantities of saliva on their coats by licking themselves clean.
The saliva dries on the hair and eventually becomes airborne.
Like saliva, drops of urine can dry on portions of the haircoat
or skin and also cause trouble.

Treatments

There are three medical approaches to treating allergies: 1) The symptoms may be controlled with various medications, in the form of pills, creams, inhalers, etc. 2) The allergic responses in the body can be lowered (sometimes eliminated) with *desensitizing* injections, which are given over a long period of time. They introduce low doses of the allergen into the body. Those allergic to cats are particularly responsive to this form of treatment. It is felt by some experts that approximately one third of patients receiving full-term desensitization have complete, permanent relief from their symptoms. Another third have a recurrence in one year and the rest in five to fifteen years. 3) The most common treatment is the elimination of allergens from the patient's environment. Which means to many allergists, removing the offending pet from the house.

However, instead of throwing the cat away, an allergy patient could try a multifaceted approach to the problem that has been encouraged by various humane groups and accepted by some allergists.

Reducing Allergy Symptoms
Without Trashing the Cat

First, find an allergist sensitive to your feelings for your pet. Second, invest in a large, commercial-size air purifier for your *entire* living space. Be certain it is a mechanical HEPA (High Efficiency Particulate Air) purifier. If possible, have it installed in your home heating system. The National Bureau of Standards states that air filtered by a HEPA unit is free of 99.97 percent of all contaminating particles. Third, allergy-proof your home. Change to washable surfaces by eliminating as much carpeting and as many upholstered pieces and large draperies as possible. Do not accumulate stacks of old books, magazines, newspapers, and so on. Use wood or linoleum floors, washable cotton curtains, roll-up shades and blinds. Pour cat litter into the pan slowly to keep dust from rising into the air, and use a litter that is not dusty. Do not allow your cat into your bedroom. Allow your bedroom to become an allergy-free sanctuary, with the door shut. Have someone who is not allergic do the vacuuming.

And now for the good news. A commercial, nonprescription product is available to everyone to reduce or eliminate the sadness from being told you're allergic to your dog or cat. The product is called Allerpet™ and has become to pet allergies what the Salk vaccine was to polio. This highly effective product simply cleanses the animal's coat of the dander and saliva antigens of the cat. It is an important breakthrough for those who are allergic to cats.

The product is wiped onto the animal's hair coat with a wet sponge or washcloth and then brushed. Two applications for each treatment are recommended. Allerpet™ contains a combination of proteins, conditioners and collagen and is pH balanced to neutralize and reduce or eliminate dander and saliva allergens. It conditions and moisturizes pet hair and skin and restructures and seals hair shafts. It is nontoxic to pets even if they lick it. The product is not oily and will not build up on the coat. Interestingly, Allerpet™ functions as a coat conditioner, too.

This wonder product can even be used to deallergize caged pets such as ferrets, gerbils, guinea pigs, hamsters, mice, monkeys, and rabbits. It can also be useful for caged birds, although it must be applied with a fine-mist spray bottle and lightly sprayed onto the feathers. Allerpet/C is formulated for cats and the slightly stronger Allerpet/D is for dogs. They are uncomplicated, highly effective products and are useful as an addendum to most allergy therapies.

HAIRBALLS

When a cat grooms himself by licking his coat, he ingests a great deal of hair. Because the feline tongue has a spiny, abrasive surface, it pulls loose hair out of the coat when licking. The sharp-angled spines tend to catch the loose hair and keep it on the tongue until the cat eventually swallows it.

The problem is that hair is not dissolved by the digestive process and wads up into tubular-shaped ropes all along the digestive tract. These are the proverbial *hairballs*, which are not balls at all. They can eventually become a serious blockage in the stomach or intestine. Some hairballs cannot be passed from the body normally and must be removed surgically, but not without a great deal of discomfort and unpleasantness. Usually a cat will regurgitate hairballs and will have trouble keeping food down until the hair is completely out of his system.

If the cat does not regurgitate the hairball, it may move slowly down the intestine and come to a halt at some point. This will cause constipation and interfere with normal body functions. If the litter box does not have feces in it for two or three days, the cat is constipated. Constipation caused by hairballs is a serious condition and must be relieved quickly. It can cause a life-threatening problem if the blockage occurs between the stomach and the bowel.

Brushing and combing your cat every day will definitely help prevent this problem. An abundance of hairball remedies are available in most pet supply stores and mail-order catalogs. They are made mostly of malt-flavored petroleum jelly and effectively solve the problem, providing it has not been allowed to go on too long.

PREVENTION

Some pets are in the vet's office on a revolving-door basis with far too many ailments, while others go once a year, just for a checkup. If your dog or cat is on the sick list too much, it may be something you're *not* doing. Here are some guidelines that will give you and your pet a shot at good health based on prevention.

Preventive medicine can be stored into several categories. These represent good pet care and can be highly effective for maintaining good health.

Vaccinations

Many infectious diseases are prevented through the use of vaccines. No vaccine is 100 percent successful, but an intelligent vaccination schedule, administered by a health professional, allows kittens and mature cats the best chance for escape from serious diseases, many of which are life-threatening.

The typical cat should be vaccinated for *Feline panleukopenia, Feline viral rhinotracheitis, Feline calicivirus, Chlamydiosis, Rabies,* and *Feline leukemia virus.* Consult your veterinarian about this. There may be differences between veterinarians based on regional conditions and medical opinions.

Nutrition

Good nutrition prevents problems. And as a pet ages, it may require a different diet or even some diet therapy. The best food is a premium commercial product that states on its label "100 percent complete" or "complete and balanced diet." These labels mean the food contains the correct proportions of nutrients that have been established by the National Academy of Science. For more information read Chapter Three, "The Eating Machine."

Grooming

There is more to grooming than meets the eye. Brushing and combing makes your pet look attractive and is essential for good hygiene, but without grooming, it is impossible to know what is going on under your pet's hair or in its ears. All cats, long- and short-haired, should be brushed daily to remove dead hair and dandruff. This not only cleans the coat and stimulates the skin, but also helps control skin ailments. Daily or even weekly grooming sessions allow the pet owner to catch significant abnormalities, such as lumps, inflammations, cuts, scratches, and even external parasites, in beginning stages. Nothing is more useful than frequent home examinations.

Other important aspects of grooming and hygiene are baths, nail clipping, eye and ear hygiene, and investigation of various body odors. Refer to Chapter Six, "A Good-Looking Cat."

Dental Care

Much dental work performed by veterinarians would be unnecessary if proper care were taken by the owner. Tartar accumulates constantly in a dog or cat's mouth and should be removed on a regular basis to prevent mouth odor, gum disease, and loss of teeth. Clean your cat's teeth once a week, or more, with a soft toothbrush or cotton swab dipped in a paste of warm water and table salt or baking soda. This will save you costly vet bills and avoid the use of anesthesia when removing tartar buildup. Do not use toothpaste formulated for humans.

Exercise

The relationship between exercise and good health for pets is the same as it is for humans. Most cats give themselves a daily physical workout until they get older. This usually takes place late at night, when they get the "crazies," an energy spill where they run back and forth, pretending to stalk, ambush, and pounce on an imaginary mouse. Do not rely on this alone for your cat's exercise. Play with him, using a ball, a rubber toy, a peacock feather, or even a crumpled piece of paper. Cats enjoy anything that arouses their hunting behavior. A piece of string dangled up and down is like a bird or flying insect. A Ping-Pong ball in an empty tissue box is like a mouse on the loose. Exercise can be fun for you and your pet. It can also promote good health.

Mental Well-Being

Emotional stress can shorten a pet's life as surely as any disease. Anxiety can bring about various forms of physical stress. However, it is not difficult to promote anxiety-free conditions for your cat. Routines, habits, and established behavior patterns should be respected and maintained where possible. Play games and talk to your pet. Touch him when expressing affection. Teach your cat a trick or two, if you can. Try not to separate him from his home or his family. Do not holler at him, and never hit him.

Medical Care

Have your cat examined by a veterinarian at least once a year, more if the animal is old. Watch for signs of illness and do not wait before seeing the doctor—early treatment sometimes avoids life-threatening disease. When your cat is not acting like himself, call your vet for advice.

HOT WEATHER TIPS

- Do not shave off your pet's long-haired coat in the summer. It provides protection against heat and insects. A long coat can actually insulate a cat from the heat. A clean, brushed coat helps prevent skin problems, too.
- Keep your cat out of parked cars. A car turns quickly into an oven in warm weather and causes life-threatening heat prostration. This is true even if the windows are slightly open and the car is parked in the shade. Do not allow your cat to lick antifreeze or auto coolants. They are highly toxic and life-threatening for small animals.
- When traveling long distances with your cat, it is best to drive in the early morning and late afternoon hours, when it is cooler. Provide your cat with plenty of cool, clean water. Carry a gallon thermos filled with cold water and ice.
- Keep your cat in cool, shady areas during hot, humid weather. Bring your cat inside where it is cool and shady.
- Be on the lookout for fleas and ticks. Because of the various diseases associated with these parasites, see a veterinarian at the first signs, which include intense scratching and nipping of the skin, in addition to pawing at the head.

COLD WEATHER TIPS

- Keep your cat inside. Outdoor cats can easily freeze, become lost, be stolen, get hurt, or even die, under the wheels of a skidding car.
- Never leave your cat alone in a car during cold weather. A car can become like a refrigerator in the winter, holding in the cold. Your cat could freeze to death.
- Increase your cat's food ration in the winter *if* he is not obese and is in a normal state of health. This will help him to maintain his normal energy level and protect his thick hair coat throughout the winter season. Consult your veterinarian about added amounts to feed.
- Do not allow your cat to sleep in drafty areas. Keep him off the floor, if possible. Provide him with a cozy cat bed with a warm blanket in it and place it on a level higher than the floor.
- Before starting up your car (in or out of your garage), check to see if your cat is under the hood, next to the engine, where it is warm.

POISONOUS PLANTS

Nature is a harsh mother when pet meets plant. If a cat jumps into a rosebush, it's bad for the roses, but it's worse for the cat. It is a thorny problem. A shorthaired cat walking through a patch of nettles is on shaky ground, as he will probably have tremors and twitches by the end of the day. When our beloved fauna tries to eat our beloved flora, the flora sometimes fights back. Whether your cat is indoors or outdoors, he is vulnerable to the harmful effects of some plants.

What do *Japanese yew, mountain laurel, lily of the valley, philodendron, and dieffenbachia* all have in common? They are beautiful to look at but potentially toxic to pets, children, and even to ourselves. Although plant poisoning is uncommon, small animals and young children can find themselves in a life-threatening emergency if they nibble on plants such as these.

However, it would be a great disservice to those who love the refreshing beauty of natural greenery to advise them to ban *all* such plants from their homes. Instead, it is useful to know which plants are potentially harmful, in order to prevent accidents. Toxic plants only produce the effects of poisoning after sufficient quantities have been eaten. The toxic dosage varies with the species of plant, the stage of plant growth, the part of the plant consumed, the soil type, and other environmental factors. The animal species also affects dosages; dogs may be more susceptible to a given plant poison than cats or birds.

It is fortunate that dogs and cats do not depend on foliage as a staple in their diet. In most situations, they will eat only a small quantity of the offending growth, with little or no reaction to it. Of course, almost all outdoor cats eat grass and then regurgitate it. Some believe this behavior relates to the animal's need or desire to cleanse its digestive tract. Pets that nibble away at plants usually do so out of boredom or curiosity. Other factors involved in plant eating are the age of the animal, the feeding habits of the owner, and new or altered surroundings. Although kittens are less likely than adult cats to eat foreign materials such as plants, they will on occasion be tempted by them.

Teething irritation may be relieved by chewing on objects in the environment. Any available plant materials, such as seeds, pits, bulbs, branches, and even leaves, may be chewed and ingested. Make the surroundings safe for young or old cats by removing or preventing access to hazardous substances, including toxic plants.

Poisonous plants may affect the mouth, throat, esophagus, stomach, intestines, nervous system, blood and circulation, heart, or brain (altered behavior, hallucinations). The signs may be mild, such as lack of energy, or intense, involving digestive upsets, or extreme, involving depression, coma, and death. When such signs are apparent, it is important to consider plant poisoning as a possibility if the animal has been exposed to toxic growths.

Poisonous plants affecting the mouth, throat, and esophagus with irritation, ulcers, excessive salivation, or swelling (sometimes interfering with breathing) are dumb cane, philodendron, caladium, skunk cabbage, and jack in the pulpit. Plants affecting the stomach and digestive tract with either irritation, vomiting, nausea, depression, abdominal pain, diarrhea, possible fever, coma, or death are amaryllis, daffodil, tulip, and wisteria bulbs; English ivy; alfalfa; beech; daphne; iris; bird of paradise; box; crown of thorns; euonymus; honeysuckle; poinsettia; castor bean; precatory bean (rosary pea); black locust; nightshades; Jerusalem cherry; and potato (green parts and eyes).

Those affecting the cardiovascular system are foxglove, lily of the valley, oleander, monkshood, larkspur, cherry pits, peach pits, apricot pits, almond pits, apple seeds, and hydrangea.

Plants affecting the nervous system with either trembling, irregular heartbeat, abdominal pain, nausea, vomiting, salivation, convulsions, thirst, alterations in behavior, dilated pupils, or sudden death are Japanese yew, English yew, Western yew, American yew, Indian tobacco, golden chain, mescal bean, poison hemlock, tobacco, rhubarb (leaves, upperstem), belladonna, henbane, jimson weed, jessamine, datura, periwinkle, chinaberry, coriaria, moonseed, water hemlock, marijuana, and morning glory.

Among dangerous plants, the least considered or understood are those that are "mechanically injurious," those plants that either irritate, lacerate, or puncture the skin, or injure the body by physical force. Contact irritants or mechanical injuries can be produced by nettle, nettle spurge, stinging nettle, bull nettle, burdock, blackberry, cactus, Carolina nightshade, foxtail, goathead, honey locust, needlegrass, sandbur, tripleawn, wild barleys, and wild bromes.

The list of plants potentially dangerous to pets is, indeed, a long one. A few general principles should be remembered. First, get the poisonous material out of the animal by inducing vomiting, usually. Take the plant away if the animal is "caught in the act." Contact a veterinarian immediately for instructions.

The most important element of plant poisoning is prevention. Keep poisonous plants hanging out of your pet's reach, or in a separate room that is off-limits to cats. As the spring gardening season approaches, bear in mind that outdoor plants can carry chemical poisons. Highly toxic herbicides and organophosphate pesticides on grass clippings can also be deadly.

When plant poisoning does occur, it may be a life-threatening situation requiring fast action if your pet is to survive. Take the following action: 1) Try to determine what the poisonous material was, when it was eaten, and the amount swallowed. 2) Call your veterinarian or nearest poison control center. Inform your veterinarian of your cat's age, any medical problems, if he is taking medication, and whether or not he has vomited. 3) If possible, bring the poisonous material to the veterinarian with the cat. The sooner you get professional advice, the better the chance for survival. Remember, plant poisoning is rare, but poisonous plants are not.

BIRTH CONTROL

Anyone who has ever loved a cat will be appalled to know that millions of cats are abandoned and impounded every year. Of these unwanted, helpless creatures, 90 percent are destroyed. The effect is morally and psychologically poisonous. The fact is that there are more cats in the world than there are homes for them, even though 50 million families live with one or more cats. But those who have ever tried to find a taker for a kitten or grown cat know that there are not enough homes to go around.

In light of all this, birth control becomes a vitally important issue. That's a term not usually applied to pets, but any loving cat owner will recognize it as the only way to curtail a burgeoning population of unwanted animals and all its attendant woes.

Probably the most important and effective form of pet birth control is surgical sterilization. In the female this is referred to as *spaying* or *ovariohysterectomy* and involves the removal of the animal's ovaries and related reproductive organs. For male cats the procedure is referred to as *neutering* or *castration*. Cats that have been surgically sterilized are referred to as *altered* or *fixed*.

Contrary to popular belief, altered cats do not become fat, nor do they lose their personalities, although altered males lose some of their aggressiveness and other nasty traits.

There is another form of birth control, but it applies only to female cats and must be obtained from a veterinarian. It is a prescription drug that functions in much the same manner as birth control pills for humans. Consult a veterinarian as to the advisability of using this drug on your cat.

For owners of unaltered cats, eternal vigilance is one ounce of prevention. But the best preventive measure is to forestall the possibility of reproduction. The methods described are safe, humane, and responsible. If you are going to live with a cat, then do not let it reproduce, deliberately or by accident. A happy cat is one that has a home.

CHAPTER EIGHT

The Sick Cat

MEDICAL SIGNS OF ILLNESS

It is not always easy to know when to take your cat to a veterinarian. In addition to annual checkups and vaccinations, your cat may need medical diagnosis and treatment for any one of dozens of ailments that befall the average pet, ranging from minor to gravely serious. To help you decide when to call and ask for help or information, here is a list of veterinary medical signs. If your cat shows one or more of these signs, call your veterinarian and ask for an opinion.

Depression
Low, throaty crying
Bladder enlargement
Cloudy urine
Pink urine
Red urine
Extremely yellow urine
Constant straining to urinate
   resulting in small dribbles
   both in and out of the litter box
Inability to urinate
Constant leaking of urine
Pale gums
Change in eating habits:
   Difficulty eating
   Increased appetite

Poor or no appetite
Indications of poor vision
Bad breath
Vomiting (excessive)
Excessive thirst
Inability to move
Nasal discharge
Sneezing (excessive)
Drooling
Loss of hair coat
Trembling
Lumps
Hacking or coughing
Hoarseness
Loss of breath of abnormal
   breathing

Abdominal enlargement Unusual head shaking
Abdominal soreness   Diarrhea (excessive)

YOUR CAT'S DOCTOR

The front line of defense for keeping your cat healthy is first-rate medical care. As you have a family doctor, so should your cat have, a professional who is educated and trained to care for the medical needs of animals.

Veterinarians who specialize in treating pets are called *small-animal clinicians*. Small-animal medicine is a big subject that could fill volumes. After receiving bachelor degrees (or higher), students of this medicine enter veterinary colleges and continue their education for a minimum of four years. Upon graduation young veterinarians receive their doctorate degrees (D.V.M. or V.M.D.) and may serve an internship at an animal hospital before taking a state licensing examination. This is the medical education and experience that is necessary to open a veterinary practice, similar to that of any other doctor.

Sooner or later anyone with a cat will need an accredited, licensed veterinarian, because it is impossible to diagnose and treat a sick animal properly without formal medical training. However, conscientious cat owners need to know how to prevent sickness and when to see a veterinarian if they suspect their pets are sick.

Some cats frequent the vet's office on a revolving-door basis with far too many ailments, while others go once a year for a checkup or even less often. If your cat seems to be forever on the sick list, it may be something you're *not* doing. The most important thing you can do for your cat's health is see a veterinarian at least once a year for an annual checkup.

THE VETERINARY EXAMINATION

Cats require a physical examination by a veterinarian at least once a year. Vaccinations must also be boosted from time to time, usually every year. But few pet owners really know what's happening during the annual checkup, and whether or not the animal is getting a thorough examination. Here is an example of what a good physical examination of your cat should consist of, with guidelines provided by the American Animal Hospital Association, which is an organization of veterinarians who have a special commitment to the quality of small-animal medicine.

Eyes

An animal's eyes reflect many facts about its health. Anemia, infections, and jaundice may be discovered by eye examinations. Some breeds of cats have eye disorders that are commonly seen at birth. Veterinarians are trained in early detection of these conditions. An animal's eyes are also subject to ulcers and injury. Vets use an instrument called an *ophthalmoscope* to observe the inner structure of the eyes, especially the lens and retina. It is an instrument containing a perforated mirror and lenses. The doctor will look for cataracts in older cats, as well as cloudy lenses or other symptoms of disease, with the help of the ophthalmoscope.

Ears

Cats have deep, curved ear canals which provide protection for the inner ear but which, unfortunately, also provide a nesting place for infection and disease. Ear infection is common in cats and can often be detected by a foul odor in the ear or by the animal's tendency to shake and scratch its head. To properly examine the ear canal, the veterinarian uses an instrument called an *otoscope*, a tubular flashlight with a funnel at the end that is inserted into the cat's ear canal. By looking into the wide end of the funnel, he or she can get a better view of the ear canal and the organs within it. The vet will usually check all parts of the ear and ear flap for parasites, ulcers, infections, and foreign matter.

Nose

A cat's nose is not the health barometer most people believe it to be. A healthy animal's nose may be hot or cold, wet or dry. The veterinarian will check your cat's nose for discharges or other irregularities. He or she may also use a light to examine the nasal passages for any weed seeds or plant particles that have lodged there.

Mouth

The condition of an animal's gums, tongue, and palate is closely observed. The color of the lining of the lips and gums is particularly important. The lack of a pink or red color in this area could indicate anemia. The veterinarian will also check the mouth area for tumors, ulcers, and other abnormalities.

Teeth

Oral hygiene is as important to pets as it is to humans, and should not be overlooked. Kittens may need help to remove "milk" or baby teeth. Many vets today use ultrasonic and other types of equipment that are the same or very similar to those used in human dentistry. But, unlike humans, most pets require sedation or anesthesia for thorough dental treatment.

Respiratory System

The vet's examination of the mouth area will continue with an evaluation of the larynx (or voice box) and trachea, which is the pathway to the lungs. A *stethoscope*, which magnifies the sounds of the lungs, will be used as part of the screening process. The results of this screening will determine if further examinations or tests are required.

Spine/Musculoskeletal

If possible, your cat's gait or walk should be observed to spot any abnormalities of the pelvis. Using his or her sense of touch, a veterinarian will examine the cat's neck, dorsum (backbone), and tail. The fleshy fat covering any muscle tone will be evaluated as part of the screening process.

Skin

The skin is the largest organ of the body. Its condition and that of the cat's hair coat are important health indicators. Part of the examination of the skin will include looking for evidence of fleas, ticks, and other parasites; tumors; wounds; and infections. The lymph nodes under the skin should also be checked. Some skin conditions require skin scrapings, tissue biopsies, or allergy tests to identify the problem. Laboratory analysis may be necessary.

Legs

The vet should use his or her eyes and sense of touch to examine the cat's limbs. Close attention should be paid to the cat's joints—for possible deformation, inflammation or disease. The doctor should also closely check the feet and foot pads for any inflammation, deformities or embedded matter.

Reproductive System

A thorough physical for your cat should include a careful examination of the reproductive system for abnormalities. Most pet cats are spayed (females) or neutered (males) for reasons other than birth control. For example, neutering of male cats reduces the incidence of prostate disease and some types of cancer. Neutering may also help eliminate or modify some behavioral problems such as aggressiveness or the tendency to roam. Spaying (*ovariohysterectomy*) eliminates the possibility of a serious uterine infection (*pyometra*). Ovario-hysterectomy may also reduce or eliminate the incidence of breast cancer if completed before the first "heat" (*estrus*).

Abdominal Cavity

The doctor should use his or her hands to press, touch, and feel the abdomen for any excess fluids, gas, or tumors. The spleen, bladder, kidneys, intestines, and liver should also be evaluated. A male cat's enlarged prostate gland or a female's enlarged uterus, as well as other abnormalities, may be detected as part of the abdominal cavity screening examination.

Cardiovascular System

A stethoscope will be used to evaluate the heart. Any abnormal sounds or beats may lead to additional tests, such as X rays and electrocardiograms (ECGs). Radiographs (X rays) are important diagnostic tools. As a matter of record, the American Animal Hospital Association not only requires that hospital members of their association have a separate facility for radiology, but that the vet produce high-quality X-ray films.

Anal Area

Rubbing the haunches, or "scooting," generally indicates an anal sac problem. Cats have such sacs on each side of the anal opening, and they may become enlarged or infected. Sometimes the condition is referred to as "impacted anal glands." The veterinarian should be able to easily identify and treat this problem, and also note and evaluate any tumors that may be present.

Vaccinations

Probably the most important reason for your cat's annual checkup is to give him his annual booster shots for added medical protection. One of the greatest advances in helping animals live longer, more comfortable lives is the highly effective vaccinations against life-threatening diseases. Many inoculations are now given in one multiple injection to prevent several disease threats at the same time.

Most veterinarians recommend early vaccination of kittens, and then a series of booster shots. You are then asked to bring the animal in once a year for added protection. Which vaccinations are recommended and their schedules sometimes vary from one veterinarian to another. The program used in catteries may be different from the one recommended for cats in the home. Veterinarians are aware of local disease problems and will tailor specific vaccination recommendations and programs to their geographical area. Typical recommendations may include immunization of cats against feline panleukopenia, feline viral rhinotracheitis, feline calicivirus, chlamydiosis, rabies, and feline leukemia virus.

An annual physical examination for your cat is no longer a novelty. For the concerned animal lover it is an absolute necessity. Selecting the right veterinarian and then trying to understand his or her procedures is the responsibility of the human caretaker. With this accomplished, it is then important to follow the advice of the veterinarian. With the proper medication and medical treatment, both humans and animals can live more comfortable and longer lives. Today, a cat can enjoy much of the same high caliber of medical services that is available to his human family. You need only seek it out.

SERIOUS INFECTIOUS DISEASES OF THE CAT

Cats, like all living beings, are vulnerable to many diseases. Some of them are cured by the immune system; some are not. It is helpful to all cat owners to be aware of the major feline illnesses, if only to understand what a veterinarian is trying to tell them. Although cat owners are often unable to do anything on their own to stop the ravages of a major disease once it has been established, it is important to be able to recognize the signs as they occur. This helps you take the proper action which, of course, is to see a veterinarian. *The following major diseases are, for the most part, preventable by vaccinations.*

Rabies

Rabies is probably the most notorious yet least understood viral disease of all warm-blooded animals. To understand rabies one must understand the nature of a virus. A virus is a microorganism so small that only the most powerful electronic microscope can actually see it. It is a life form that multiplies profoundly once it has settled into a host organism. Parasitic in nature, it has no mechanism for providing energy for its own reproduction. Therefore, it must enter the cells of other living organisms and use the energy and material of those cells to feed its own drive to replicate. This is biological theft and kills the cells the virus robs, causing damage, injury, and in some cases death, to the host organism.

Rabies is a fatal virus, an acute infectious disease of the central nervous system. The virus enters the body and travels to nerve endings. Over a period of time it moves to the spinal cord and eventually makes its way to the brain, where it causes eventual degeneration of the entire nervous system. It produces altered behavior, paralysis, and death.

The usual mode of transmission is through a bite from an animal carrying the virus in its saliva. The rabies virus can also enter the body through contact with an open wound or scratch, although this is less common.

The incubation period between entry of the virus into the body and the first signs of the disease varies, from one week to one year. This is determined by how long the virus remains within the muscle cells at the site of the bite, before it is able to get to the central nervous system. Once it makes its way to nerve endings, it is able to reach the spinal cord within four to five days, and then to travel persistently upward until it ultimately reaches the brain. From there it spreads to other parts of the body, including the salivary glands, the respiratory system, and the digestive tract. During this period it can be transmitted to another animal by biting, because of its involvement with the host's saliva.

The disease is seen in cats in two stages, each showing its own signs. The first stage is an excitatory, or "furious," stage; the second, a paralytic, or "dumb," stage. An infected cat will probably experience some indications of both stages.

The "furious" stage may last from one to seven days and is marked by seemingly wild and aggressive behavior. The cat becomes extremely dangerous because of its desire to bite and the speed with which it can bite anyone or anything nearby.

Drooling and difficulty in swallowing are also characteristic of this phase.

The paralytic or "dumb" stage may last for only one or two days. It is the final stage of the disease, if death does not come sooner. The paralysis first appears in the muscles of the head and neck; the lower jaw hangs open and the cat cannot eat or drink. Localized paralysis shortly becomes generalized throughout the body, with death resulting in one or two days.

Rabies is a fatal disease for those infected, including small animals and humans. In North America rabies is most frequently carried by infected skunks, raccoons, foxes, bats, and other animals living in the wild. A wild animal that allows you to get close to it is behaving in an uncharacteristic manner and may have rabies. It should be avoided. If you have the slightest suspicion that your pet has been bitten by a rabid animal, you must exercise the utmost care to avoid being bitten. Report the incident to your veterinarian, your doctor, and to the health authorities in your community. Do not go near the animal, do not touch it, and confine it in isolation as quickly as possible. If you have been bitten by any animal, clean the wound thoroughly with soap and hot water and see a doctor quickly.

Because there is no cure for rabies, every cat must be vaccinated to avoid this gruesome disease. There are now vaccines available that will give your cat immunity for several years. Some animal professionals, such as dog trainers, are also being vaccinated.

Feline Panleukopenia (FPL)

This dreaded disease is also known as *feline distemper* or *feline infectious enteritis*. It is the most devastating disease affecting unvaccinated cats. It results in a high death rate, particularly among kittens and older cats. Older cats that do recover may never quite regain their health. Cats become infected by either direct or indirect contact with the disease. Studies have shown that households inhabited by sick animals can remain infective for over a year.

Temperature increases from slight to extreme (from 102°F to

104°F) are common a few days before such outward signs as loss of appetite and depression appear. This usually is followed by thirst, with a fear of drinking; vomiting of watery, yellow liquid; and either diarrhea (sometimes bloody) or constipation. As the disease progresses, the animal becomes dehydrated. Panleukopenia is carried by the air and may be caught by a cat's breathing it in from infected cats. Infected cats also spread it through their excrement, urine, and nasal discharge. One cat easily infects many others. All cats should be vaccinated for this disease starting when they're kittens, in their eighth week and again four weeks later. In high-risk areas a third vaccination should be given at sixteen weeks of age.

Feline Respiratory Diseases

Feline respiratory disease is not one disease, but a generic term for several different ones, all of which produce similar signs in the cat. Typical infections produce an unsightly and debilitating condition. All feline respiratory diseases are characterized by sneezing, tearing, inflammation of the eyes and nose, and ocular and nasal discharge. (These may be signs of other illnesses as well.) Affected cats lose weight and become vulnerable to additional infections. Death can occur, especially among young kittens, pregnant females, and older cats. The various types of feline respiratory disease result from infection by different microorganisms. Each disease has unique characteristics.

Rhinotracheitis (FVR). This is an acute respiratory disease of cats caused by a herpes virus. From 30 to 40 percent of feline respiratory disease is attributable to it. The first evidence of illness includes sneezing, elevated temperature, drooling, and depression. Other signs are heavy discharge from the eyes and nose, ulcerated tongue, rough and soiled hair coat, failure to eat, and mouth breathing due to plugged nasal passages. If uncomplicated, the disease may run its course in one to two weeks. Rhinotracheitis has a 50 percent death rate among kittens, but few grown cats die from the infection.

Calicivirus (FCV). This is another acute respiratory disease infection. It not only infects the respiratory tract, but also membranes of the mouth, causing painful tongue ulcers. Mild salivation and nasal discharge may occur. Because of the painful oral ulcers, affected cats often refuse to eat. Generally these conditions persist for two to three days; then the animal recovers without treatment.

Feline chlamydiosis *(Pneumonitis).* This respiratory disease is more related to a bacteria than to a virus. The first sign of the disease is a slight rise in body temperature. This is followed by watering of the eyes, then a slight discharge from the nose. Sneezing and coughing, although rare, may occur. Frequently the disease persists for extended periods, and recurrent infections are common. Few kittens or cats die from it.

Feline infectious peritonitis *(FIP).* FIP is not normally included in the respiratory disease complex, but it does affect the respiratory system and therefore appears in this section. FIP is a disease of cats that is difficult (sometimes impossible) to diagnose, much less treat. It is a fatal illness for cats.

This complex infection has two principal forms. In the *effusive* or wet form a rapid development ensues resulting in fluid in one or more body cavities. The abdominal cavity enlarges until the abdomen swells. If the fluid accumulation occurs in the chest cavity, it compresses the lungs, releasing fluid into the airways. It is the more severe, shorter form of the disease, almost always ending in death. The *noneffusive* or dry form is the more insidious of the two, causing failure of the kidneys, the liver, the pancreas, and other internal systems, and resulting in a gradual breakdown of body functions and eventual death.

FIP is a severe, usually fatal, generalized disease of cats caused by a coronavirus. It tends to infect cats between three and four years of age. Initially, the virus may enter through and grow in the respiratory system. Complicating matters to a great degree is its relationship to the immune system. It is suspected that antibodies contribute to the disease rather than provide protection. FIP can be spread from one cat to another, but the mode of transmission is still unverified. Most likely the infection is spread through ingestion or inhalation. It is caused by a virus that is related to other viruses which include *feline enteric coronavirus (FECV), canine coronavirus (CCV),* and the swine agent, *transmissible gastroenteritis virus (TGEV).*

Feline infectious peritonitis may take as long as five months to produce signs after the initial infection. Loss of appetite, high fever, weakness, and inflammation of the linings of the chest and abdominal cavities are the principal symptoms. When fluid accumulates, the abdomen begins to swell, as does the chest cavity.

FIP was first reported in 1966. Although much is understood about this fatal disease, there is still much to be learned, and intense research continues in an effort to develop an effective vaccine against it.

All of these diseases attacking the respiratory system may occur simultaneously, complicating diagnosis and making recovery even more difficult. Of the four diseases, only feline chlamydiosis (pneumonitis) can be treated once infection has developed. Since rhinotracheitis, calicivirus, and feline infectious peritonitis are viral diseases, they do not respond to antibiotics. Cats can be vaccinated against all of these infectious respiratory diseases listed here with the exception of feline infectious peritonitis.

Feline Immunodeficiency Virus (FIV)

It is only recently that FIV was isolated and characterized as the feline equivalent to AIDS or HIV in humans. Although FIV is related to feline leukemia virus, it does *not* cause cancer. FIV is suspected of being transmitted through saliva; therefore bite wounds are of particular concern, along with shared food and water bowls in multiple cat households. Interestingly, it is thought *not* to be transmitted through sexual contact or through pregnancy, making it quite different from HIV (AIDS).

FIV is a retrovirus of the lentivirus subfamily. When the virus infects a cell, it carries with it a special enzyme, reverse transcriptase, which is inserted into the host cell. This changes the genetic coding and allows the virus to remain in an inactive state for some time before production of new viruses is initiated. In more technical terms the virus starts out as a single-stranded RNA (ribonucleic acid). The virus then produces a double-stranded DNA (deoxyribonucleic acid) copy of the RNA. The double-stranded copy is then inserted into the DNA of the host cell, thus allowing the copy to reproduce. What makes the infection so dangerous is that antibodies within the cat do not bind to or attack this particular virus, which is similar to feline leukemia virus in this respect.

At this time FIV is considered by some researchers to be a disease of older cats. Its incubation period may be as long as three years. Clinical signs may include neurological disorders; anemia; swollen lymph glands; 103°F fever or higher; loss of appetite; severe weight loss (wasting); infections of the gums, mouth, skin, urinary bladder, upper respiratory tract, intestinal tract (causing persistent diarrhea); reproductive failures (involuntary abortion), seizures, mental deterioration, and other neurologic disorders.

Diagnosis is based on medical history, clinical signs, and the result of an FIV antibody test, which is available in kit form for use in private veterinary practices. A positive test result indicates the cat is infected with FIV and is capable of transmitting it to other cats. The cats at highest risk are free-roaming cats and those in multiple cat households where one cat is FIV positive.

Treatment consists of traditional therapies for the secondary infections for long periods of time. These involve antibiotic or antifungal drugs, intravenous fluids, blood transfusions, dietary supplements, corticosteroids (or other anti-inflammatory drugs), and anabolic steroids. There is no therapy currently available to treat the FIV infection itself, and a possible vaccine is a long way from reality at this writing. However, the incidence of FIV in catteries is very low. Indoor cats and those that do not come in contact with free-roaming cats are unlikely to contract the FIV infection. If one cat in a multiple cat household tests positive, it must be removed or isolated from the others. All cats in a multiple cat household should be tested.

Feline Leukemia Virus (FeLV)

Feline leukemia virus is one of the most serious, if not the most serious, of the fatal cat diseases because of its unique ability to insert its own genetic code into infected cells and promote permanent, long-term infection. The group of viruses with this ability are called *retroviruses*. FeLV causes leukemia (cancer of white blood cells) and lymphosarcoma (cancer of lymph tissue cells) in cats. It is a highly contagious virus that is transmitted among cats in a manner similar to other respiratory viruses. Saliva appears to be the most important vehicle for virus transmission from cat to cat, and infection involves relatively close contact between cats. Transmission is also suspected from the social grooming habits of infected cats, licking and biting, sneezing, and sharing of litter boxes and feeding bowls. Infected queens may also pass the virus on to fetuses across the placenta and to newborn kittens through the colostrum and milk.

Infected cats are subject to development of a number of diseases that are either directly or indirectly caused by FeLV. Included among them are lymphosarcoma, various forms of anemia, kidney disease, various reproductive disorders, destruction of the thymus, and a breakdown of the immune system.

There are two possible outcomes once a cat is diagnosed with FeLV. First, the cat may be able to control the infection and produce antibodies to kill the viruses. These cats successfully develop immunity to the leukemia virus and do not get leukemia or other diseases caused by the virus.

The second possible outcome is that the cat's immune system will be overcome by the virus and will not be able to limit its growth. In this event, FeLV will establish an active and persistent infection within the cat's body. Once established, it will persist for the remainder of the cat's life. Such cats may not show any signs of illness for years, but the virus will be present in their saliva, urine, and feces, and thereby infect other cats.

The percentage of cats that recover from this disease is small. Currently, there are no successful treatments for elimination of FeLV infection or the leukemia it causes, although a variety of chemotherapeutic regimens have been developed to produce a temporary remission. These are not cures, and only the symptoms can be treated, with the hope of prolonging life.

Infected cats must be identified and removed from contact with other cats. Currently, there are two types of blood tests in common use for positive diagnoses: the *enzyme-linked immunosorbent assay* (ELISA, or kit) test, which can be performed in the veterinarian's office, and the *immunofluorescence assay* (IFA, Hardy, or slide) test, which must be sent out to a diagnostic laboratory. In some instances the one test may read positive, while the other reads negative on the same cat. It is subject to interpretation by the veterinarian.

There are vaccines currently available for the prevention of FeLV infection. There are also complex pros and cons to vaccinating for this terminal illness. It is a matter of personal choice after serious consultation with a veterinarian.

Anemia

Signs of anemia are fever, depression, loss of appetite, weakness, emaciation, and jaundice. The disease can be induced through a microscopic parasite that attacks red blood cells, destroying them, and causing internal bleeding and infection. It may also result from internal or external parasite attack. Anemia results from the loss of healthy red blood cells.

Reasonably healthy cats are able to rid themselves of this disease when they are treated by a veterinarian. Cat owners must be vigilant and watch for signs of anemia so the disease does not pass from a latent form to an active state.

Lyme Disease

Lyme disease, like leptospirosis, is an infection caused by a corkscrew-shaped bacteria known as a spirochete. It is a serious condition that does not confine itself to one area within the infected body. It begins with a simple tick bite, but if untreated, it spreads to the nervous system, the heart, and the joints. It is transmitted to animals and humans by the bite of the tiny deer tick or the bear tick. The greatest chance of becoming infected is May through September, which is the period of greatest activity for these ticks in their nymphal stage.

This debilitating disease was first identified in Lyme, Connecticut, in 1975 but has since spread to many parts of North America. Although it was once thought to be found exclusively in wooded areas and grasslands, it has spread to lawns, grassy fields, and cow and horse pastures.

The disease is difficult to detect in cats because of the lack of definite signs. The problem is that animals rarely develop the initial rash that is found on infected humans. Clinical signs are elevated fever, falling off of appetite, and lameness where there was never a history of lameness and no other apparent reason for it. These signs appear several weeks after the tick bite. Within months other signs appear, such as off and on lameness, swollen lymph nodes, inflammation of the kidneys, and inflammation within the walls of the heart. The cat may also experience weight loss. Proper diagnosis is difficult and only possible with a recent medical history of signs and by laboratory blood tests. Although there are treatments involving antibiotics offering relief from pain and lameness, they must be administered early in the progression of the disease. Otherwise, treatment is prolonged, with a slower response to it.

Prevention is the best therapy. Avoidance of areas where ticks are known to be is the primary prevention. The chances of contracting Lyme disease are much less if your cat is kept indoors, where deer ticks are less likely to be found. If your cat is allowed outdoors, examine his body continually for the presence of ticks. Remove the tick quickly and efficiently if one has taken hold. Use a quality tick repellent on your cat as a preventive measure (ask a veterinarian). If your cat has a tick on its body, take hold of it with a small tweezers and pull it straight out. Try to avoid leaving any part under the skin. Apply an antiseptic to the bitten area. Destroy the tick by soaking it in alcohol. Save it and note the date it was found on the body; if signs appear, the identification of the tick is useful. See a veterinarian for an examination, blood test, and possible treatment. It is important to know that it is mandatory to report cases of Lyme disease in most states throughout the country.

Feline Urologic Syndrome (FUS)

Although many cat owners refer to this disease by such names as cystitis and urinary obstruction, FUS is not a series of interchangeable terms. FUS is an overall term for several related medical conditions located in the lower urinary tract of mostly male and some female cats. These conditions are often interconnected, although they may appear individually. FUS involves inflammation of the urinary bladder and urethra and the formation of urinary stones and plugs that cause obstruction of the urethra. Signs of this condition are frequent attempts to urinate, straining, and possibly traces of blood in the urine. Immediate medical attention is necessary.

FUS consists of *cystitis, urolithiasis,* and *urethral obstruction.* There is some disagreement among researchers and other health professionals as to the cause of this painful condition that can be life-threatening if not treated promptly. Consult with your veterinarian about this condition seen frequently, particularly in male cats. Most cats suffering from FUS not only survive, but respond well to treatment, although there is a small percentage of deaths. In chronic, recurring cases, surgery may be recommended.

Urolithiasis. The formation of stones or hardened solids in the urinary tract and the medical problems associated with them. The stones are promoted by a combination of factors including urine that is concentrated and retained by the cat for prolonged periods of time, and the excessive presence of various substances that may or may not be a result of dietary imbalance.

In many cases, the stones that are formed in the bladder pass through without incident. However, some may accumulate in the urethra of the male cat if it is too narrow a passage. The stones may be formed in the kidneys (rarely), ureters (connective ducts between the kidneys and the bladder), the bladder, or the urethra. The stones are composed primarily of magnesium ammonium phosphate or *struvite*. The troubling *urethral plug,* found in the male cat, is composed of crystals and other materials forming a soft, thick pulp. When a cat has urolithiasis, it may or may not develop the related medical problems associated with it. As stated before, some cats pass the stones with little incident. Those who do not will probably develop *cystitis.*

Cystitis. A bacterial infection of the bladder which in many cases is the result of *urolithiasis*. The infection will progress up the ureters to the kidneys, which is a potentially dangerous condition. Swift diagnoses and treatment are necessary. Antibiotics are usually the primary therapy. Cystitis causes damage to the interior of the bladder and creates mucus, blood, and other organic bits and pieces that may become the basis of a urethral plug.

Urethral obstruction. A blockage of the urethra, the duct through which urine is expelled from the body. In the male the urethra begins at the neck of the urinary bladder and opens at the end of the penis. In the female the urethra also begins at the urinary bladder and opens at the border between the vagina and the vaginal vestibule.

Urethral blockage occurs when the previously mentioned plugs build up in the urethral passage, slowing the outward flow of urine or stopping it altogether. Urethral obstruction in the male cat is a life-threatening emergency, and the cat owner must take quick action. The signs of this condition are frequent but unproductive attempts to urinate, with only a few drops of urine produced, which may have pink-to-red traces of blood in it, and continual licking of the penis. Other signs are irritability and restlessness and frequent urinating outside of the litter box, in various parts of the home. If the abdomen appears to be larger than usual (as large as a lemon) and is hard to the touch, it means the bladder is full and malfunctioning. Cats in this stage may cry in pain, strain constantly, vomit, and possibly drool. *This indicates an emer-*

gency situation and time is of the essence. Seek medical attention immediately. The veterinarian will have to relieve the obstruction as the first order of business. This may be accomplished by passing a catheter through the urethra and into the bladder, with the aid of a tranquilizer, sedative, or light anesthesia. Other procedures may also be necessary.

Skin Disorders

The most frequently seen medical problems of the skin are *bacterial infections.* Of these the two most common are *abscesses*, on the body, and *acne*, on and around the chin. An abscess is a pocket of infection that contains pus. The infected areas are surrounded by a membrane, much like a thick-walled balloon filled with water. An infected abscess is almost always the result of a puncture wound, a scratch, or a bite. Most of them are caused by cat fights. The winner has abscesses on the head, while the loser has them on the rear. They often require minor surgery in addition to other medical therapies.

Feline acne can develop in cats at any time during their lives, even in old age. It is the result of their not cleaning themselves properly under the chin. The symptoms are the appearance of blackheads and pimples, hair loss, and occasionally red skin and swelling. Acne does not seem to bother the cats. Gentle cleansing of the area removes many of the symptoms and can help prevent recurrences. This should be done on a regular basis with mild soap and water. Treatment is necessary when a cat starts to scratch the affected area. Most veterinarians prescribe an antibiotic for two to three weeks, with various other topical preparations. The problem tends to be a recurring one.

One of the most upsetting feline skin disorders is *ringworm,* which is not a worm or any kind of parasite. It is a fungal skin disease that causes lesions on the cat (or human), characterized by a round, hairless area with or without scales and crust formations. Usually the head and extremities are affected. The initial lesions may produce others, accompanied by broken or discolored hairs, discolored or red skin, and episodes of itchiness. As the fungus grows, it spreads out many times in circular patches on the skin surface. Ringworm is highly contagious for any mammal, including humans. Veterinary treatment and environmental management are simple but absolutely essential.

There is a dermatological syndrome known as *eczema,* which is not one specific skin disease but several. It is characterized by skin lesions with red bumps and scabs. They may be visible or may be found only by touch. They may irritate and cause scratching, licking, and hair loss, and they may exude fluids. Although eczema usually involves the back, it can spread over the surface of the entire body. Many skin diseases of undetermined cause may be attributed to eczema. More than a few laboratory tests may be necessary for a veterinarian to make a proper diagnosis and treatment.

Internal Parasites

Internal parasites are among the most common ailments of cats. Almost all kittens and adult cats get them at one time or another. For the squeamish this is one of the least pleasant subjects to confront. It is difficult for most pet owners to think that there are wormlike organisms of many species that can live within and feed off the bodies of their cats. These "worms" vary in type, size, effect, and threat to the health of the bodies they reside in. Although all worms can do harm to a cat's body, few create permanent or irreparable damage if detected and treated early enough.

Sometimes parasites produce infection or inflammation, in addition to toxic substances that harm the body. Many of these organisms ingest blood from the host animal, causing anemia and damaged tissue.

Almost all internal parasites that collect in a cat's body are called worms, with the exception of the protozoa, which are one-celled animals detectable only with a microscope. When treated promptly, the cat returns to good health. Depending on the degree of infestation, the condition runs from mild to gravely serious. It must be properly diagnosed by a veterinarian in the most specific sense and then treated medically according to type. Over-the-counter remedies are usually ineffective unless the type of worm infestation has been accurately identified.

All internal parasites produce signs that alert the cat owner to the condition, and many of these signs are similar. Early signs are lethargy, appetite loss, diarrhea, and bloody stool. The signs of heavy infestation are loss of weight, bloated stomach, dehydration, dry and thinning coat, drowsiness, and anemia.

If you suspect that your kitten or adult cat is infected, take a stool sample to your vet for diagnosis and treatment. In some instances, internal parasites do not appear in one stool, but may in others. For this reason, it is more effective to collect small specimens of from one to five stools (every other day) and bring the material to the vet for microscopic examination. Consult your veterinarian for the procedure of choice.

Roundworms (ascarids). These are long worms that can grow from three to five inches in length, are white, cylindrical in shape, and seen in the cat's stool or vomitus. Roundworms are the most common species of internal parasite found in cats. The adult worm lives in the intestine; its eggs pass from there to the stool and then out of the body. Cats may become reinfected by ingesting contaminated soil or feces, or eating prey animals that are contaminated. Ingested larvae travel through the body to the intestine and grow there to full maturity. Once again eggs are deposited in the intestine and the cycle continues.

Human infestation is possible and is particularly harmful to small children, who may be contaminated as a result of handling infested pets. A child, however, would have to ingest infested feces or rub it into a break in the skin to become infected. It is an extremely rare occurrence.

Toxocara cati, or roundworms, are most commonly transmitted in larvae from a queen to her kittens. Some of the larvae ingested by adult cats migrate to tissues of the body, where they persist for years. It is the pregnancy that reactivates them and causes migration to the mammary glands, where they are carried to the kittens in the milk.

Hookworms. Hookworms are thick, round worms that are less than an inch long and thrive in the small intestine of the adult cat. It is there that the female worm deposits thousands of eggs daily, many of which are passed on through the stool. The adults hook themselves onto the wall of the host animal's intestine and take blood meals. The result can be anemia due to severe blood loss and diarrhea due to intestinal inflammation. In the young, weak, or malnourished cat, hookworms can cause sudden collapse and death. Watch for weight loss, diarrhea, or bloody stools. The eggs are microscopic in size and cannot be specifically identified without a laboratory stool analysis.

Heartworms. Heartworms are considered to be a parasite of the dog. Still, they can infect cats through the bite of a mosquito that has previously bitten an infected animal. The worms are injected under the skin by the mosquito; from there they travel to the heart and develop into adult worms. This will eventually cause the heart to work harder to pump blood to the lungs. As the heart weakens, every other organ in the body becomes affected because of insufficient blood flow. The immature heartworms (*microfilariae*) can only be detected through laboratory analysis of blood samples. Delayed treatment results in heart failure—with or without permanent damage to the liver and kidneys—leading to death.

Treatment involves destruction of adult heartworms and elimination of the *microfilariae* from the blood. Hospitalization is almost always necessary. When *microfilariae* are present in the blood, they are relatively easy to identify, and treatment can be effective. In the dog, the larvae of heartworms may persist for years. However, cats rarely have *microfilariae* (the larval stage) in the blood for extended periods of time. Without their presence, it is difficult to determine if a cat is infected. In that case the veterinarian must rely on clinical signs, various tests for antigens or antibodies, X rays, and electrocardiograms. For this reason the disease is less commonly diagnosed in the cat.

You can protect cats from heartworms by avoiding their

exposure to the bite of mosquitoes. There is a preventative medication available for cats. However, you must not administer heartworm preventive medication unless your cat has been tested and shown to be *free* of heartworm infestation. The use of such medication should be left to the discretion of a veterinarian.

Tapeworms (cestodes). There are several types of tapeworms found in infected cats, but the most common species is the *dipylidium caninum*, which involves flea larvae as an intermediate host. The *dipylidium caninum* voids segments of its bead-like body from an infected cat from which flea larvae may feed. Another cat ingests the infected flea (usually through self grooming) and is then infected with tapeworm, thus continuing the cycle.

This parasite is known for its tenacity and indiscriminate infiltration of young and old alike. In rare cases it can be passed on to humans and requires a conscientious approach to diagnosis and treatment.

The head or *acolex* of the worm attaches itself to the intestinal lining, while the long body of segments (*proglottids*) remains free of the lining. Often the bottom segments break off and are passed in the feces, leaving the head still attached to produce new segments.

Signs of tapeworm begin with digestive upsets, irregular appetite, weight loss, stomach discomfort, and poor coat condition. Diagnosis is made by examination of the fecal matter. Look for segments of the worm in the cat's stool, bed, or anal area. At first the segments are light-colored and about a quarter-inch in length. When dry, they shrivel and turn brownish in color and granular in shape, like tiny grains of rice.

The most common source of tapeworm is fleas. Your cat also gets tapeworms by eating infected, uncooked meat, either in the wild or from the kitchen, and from raw fish. Lice can also carry the infection. Treatment involves destroying the head within the host's body. Professional medical attention from a veterinarian is essential for successful therapy.

Coccidia. This parasite is a protozoan, a simple organism composed of a single cell, and is capable of producing the medical condition known as *coccidiosis* in cats and dogs.

Coccidia infestation is extremely persistent and highly contagious to all household pets. Signs are bloody diarrhea, loss of appetite, loss of energy, dehydration, and anemia. Other indications include discharge from the eyes and nose accompanied by a persistent cough. This parasite can also be present with few or no signs at all. Several stool samples are needed for laboratory analysis in order to identify these parasites properly. They are microscopic and are transmitted through the feces of other animals. Good sanitation is important to prevent them from spreading, and veterinary treatment is vital.

Toxoplasma gondii (cause of toxoplasmosis). This parasite is a protozoan and is of great concern because of its deadly effect on the human fetus within the uterus of a pregnant woman. *Toxoplasma gondii* produces *toxoplasmosis,* a disease which is not only serious for a cat but is severely damaging or even fatal to the human fetus.

The oocysts (eggs) of *toxoplasma gondii* are passed through the feces of infected cats and require forty-eight to seventy-two hours to become infective once again. If they are eaten at the right time by another cat, the eggs settle in numerous tissues and evolve into another form known as *schizonts,* causing the disease to develop, and often continue for the life of the host animal. *Cats can become infected by eating raw meat infected with oocysts or schizonts.* Occasionally the disease is fatal to cats. It may produce fever, diarrhea, and, in some cases, generalized wasting, in which case the animal is terminal.

Adult humans in good health rarely develop disease due to infection from *toxoplasma gondii.* However, adults with immune system problems such as HIV (AIDS) or undergoing immunosuppressive therapy may experience an acute form of the disease once infected.

Fetuses that are the most seriously affected are those whose mothers are infected during the second or third trimesters of pregnancy. Prevention requires good sanitation involving urine and feces of household cats. Waste material should be disposed of frequently, but not by pregnant women. Cats must not be allowed to defecate in or near a child's play area. Cats that catch and eat mice could ingest the oocysts of toxoplasma gondii *and become a source of infection. Caution around such cats must be observed. The contents of cat litter boxes must not be used in gardens or as compost. Avoid feeding cats raw meat. Humans, especially pregnant women, can prevent infection by not eating raw or undercooked meat.*

External Parasites

Almost all cats at one time or another serve as hosts for external parasites, such as fleas, ticks, lice, and mites. They latch onto the outer body of the cat and feed from it. These tiny, sometimes microscopic, creatures damage the animal's body tissue, causing irritation and possible secondary infections. Some species take blood meals from the cat, creating a potential for anemia, while others simply bite into the skin. The annoyance, irritation, and debilitating effects of this kind of parasitic infestation can be serious, and the signs should not be taken lightly.

All external parasites can and will attach themselves to humans if given the opportunity. For this reason it is important to be observant and treat the family pet and his environment at the first sign of infestation. Check all areas where the cat is allowed, including carpets, furniture, bedding, and all the rooms, as well as every member of the household including children. If there are any signs of fleas, ticks or lice, call a professional exterminator.

Fleas. Fleas are parasites that live by taking blood meals from their host animals. Adult fleas feed only on blood. The host animal also provides a warm, compatible environment for these tormenting creatures.

Modern lifestyles, with pets living in millions of homes, have aggravated the flea problem. So have changing weather patterns and an apparent buildup of flea resistance to some standard chemical controls. It has been estimated that one mating pair of fleas, in their 274-day lifetime, can produce 222 trillion adult fleas. Fleas can cause typhus, bubonic plague, rabbit fever, tapeworm, and chronic, nonspecific dermatitis (often diagnosed as eczema).

Flea-infested cats become restless, may lose weight, and can damage their coats by biting and scratching. Cat owners may be bitten by fleas and develop skin rashes themselves. Fleas can be found anywhere in the home, in the yard, and, of course, on the animals.

In addition to the other bad effects that afflict flea-infested cats, the flea bites cause inflammation of the skin at the site of the bite. The constant scratching causes the hair to break and creates bald spots in the coat. In chronic cases, the skin thickens and becomes hard. Some cats display allergic reactions to flea bites, and the result is severe dermatitis. Large, moist patches appear in the coat, around the cat's head and neck, and on the posterior. This allergic reaction is caused by a chemical in the flea's saliva, which is introduced into the skin while the flea is sucking blood.

Cat fleas and dog fleas (actual species) have the ability to survive under the most adverse conditions. Once established, they resist all ordinary extermination efforts. Control is not difficult, but without understanding the life cycle of fleas, getting rid of them is nearly hopeless.

The adult flea has a life span of up to one year; it lays its eggs in the environment where the host animal lives—in cracks, crevices, carpeting, and so on. The eggs hatch into larvae, which remain in the environment for up to two hundred days. Each larva spins a cocoon and may remain inside it for as long as one year. Eventually it will break out of the cocoon as an adult flea and prepare to infest another animal and begin the cycle again. *The longest part of the flea's life cycle takes place in the environment and not on the cat.*

Bathing the cat with a flea shampoo or spraying the house with an aerosol bomb will get rid of adult fleas for perhaps twenty-four hours. When a few spraying operations prove unsuccessful, many cat owners conclude that the insecticide is useless, or that fleas are being brought in from an outside source. This is not necessarily true. The flea infestation is somewhere indoors. It must also be remembered that you are dealing with a colony of insects in all states of development, not just with adult fleas. Once a colony becomes established, a new supply hatches practically every day. Eggs are shed from the cat's coat wherever he goes.

During the breeding season, adult fleas are also occupied with providing flea larvae an adequate food supply. This is accomplished by a clever blood transfer system. The adult fleas draw blood from the cat in a quantity in excess of their requirements for maintenance and egg laying. This blood passes through the flea's body and is excreted in the form of minute, black crumbs which fall from the infested cat in a constant stream, providing food for the flea larvae until they reach full size, at one to three weeks. Then the young fleas spin a cocoon and remain immobile within it for at least another week or for as long as one year. This is the *pupae* stage of development. These cocoons are highly resistant to ordinary insecticidal sprays. By the time the adult flea hatches, the spray is gone.

The main problem is dealing with the steady supply of new fleas. If there is a heavy infestation, professional exterminators may be required.

The first aspect of solving the problem is to treat the cat's environment—both indoors and outdoors. Spray or dust his sleeping area with products recommended by a veterinarian or other professional. Be sure to hit the shrubs and grass where your cat likes to prowl. Apply the insecticide once a week for three weeks. Inside your home, make sure you spray deep into the crevices and bedding where your pet sleeps. If you suspect that there are fleas in your carpets, be sure to get rid of the vacuum cleaner bags after each use. Flea eggs and larvae thrive in such bags and can soon regain a foothold in your house. It's also important to spray the flea killer on carpets and then vacuum thoroughly at least three times at seven-to-ten-day intervals.

Once the environment has been treated the first time, give

the cat a bath using a flea shampoo (formulated for cats) and a dip (if recommended by your vet). A flea dip is an insecticidal product somewhat similar to a flea shampoo that is not rinsed off. It is diluted in bath water where the animal is literally dipped. It should only be used with advice from a veterinarian. Apply a flea collar or douse the cat with a good flea powder every night for a period of two to three weeks until the situation is under control. The daily use of a flea comb will help you to determine the progress of the treatment. Be careful about mixing different types of powders, sprays, chemicals, and flea collars without advice from a vet.

The most important thing to know about flea control is this: Treating your pet for fleas without simultaneously treating the environment is both inefficient and ineffective. Consult a veterinarian as well as an exterminator. Fleas are more than a nuisance. They are your cat's worst enemy.

Lice. Lice are small, black insects that live on the cat's body and take blood meals, as do fleas. The difference between lice and fleas is that fleas move from location to location on the body, while lice burrow into the skin and feed from one place. They are very small and extremely difficult to see. If the cat scratches hard, these tiny insects dig in deeper. Unlike fleas, lice lay their eggs on the cat's coat by attaching them firmly to the hairs. The lice eggs are called nits and have light-colored, waxy bodies.

Some lice live on the animal's blood while others eat loose particles of the skin. If infestation is great, the bloodsucking lice can cause considerable blood loss, hence an anemic cat. Eggs, attached to the hairs by a sticky substance, can be eliminated by a bath and an insecticidal shampoo. Consult a veterinarian and ask about secondary skin infections caused by the cat's scratching and biting.

Ticks. Ticks are parasites that feed off the blood of their hosts, robbing them of their vitality and spreading disease. The *hard tick* variety is a carrier of Rocky Mountain spotted fever, Q fever, and other, more rare diseases. The *soft tick* variety is a prolific carrier of *spirochetes*, which can cause Lyme disease.

Unlike fleas and lice, ticks are not considered insects but *arachnids*. They are in the same scientific class as spiders, scorpions, and mites. Ticks in their adult stage hunt for their final, most important blood meal from any warm-blooded creature, which often is a cat, a dog, or a human host. If they are not already established within the human environment, they wait on the blades of grass for a creature to jump on and are thus carried into the home.

There are several species of ticks that attack warm-blooded animals or simply use them to ride into the human environment. The species most frequently found is the *brown dog tick* (also known as the *American dog tick*), which is the hard tick variety. Its body is hard and flat like a thumbtack. It measures about one sixteenth of an inch in length, before feeding. When the female is engorged with the blood of the host the body may distend to a half inch. This tick can live for years inside a house with great success by infiltrating cracks, bedding, carpeting, and walls.

The life cycle of ticks is complex. They exist in four stages: egg, larva, nymph, and adult. Although they may live for years waiting for a blood meal, just a few days of their adult stage is spent on the bodies of their hosts.

Both male and female ticks inject their host and siphon blood, but it is only the female that attaches to the skin and engorges itself until it swells. The female changes color at this point from brown to gray. Mating occurs while the female is attached to the skin of the host. The male dies after copulation and drops off. The female continues to engorge itself with blood meals, swelling to proportions much greater than its original size. It then drops off, finds a suitable hiding place, lays thousands of eggs, and dies.

Within several weeks the eggs hatch into minuscule, six-legged larvae. As soon as possible, the young ticks will find a host and feed from it. The larvae detach from the host and molt into their eight-legged nymphal stage. After a feeding in this stage, the nymph becomes an adult.

To control ticks it is important to understand that they live in one place and feed in another. To rid yourself of this dangerous parasite you must treat your cat and your living environment. Use a pesticide spray formulated for ticks, both inside and outside your home. Spray the entire outer environment, paying particular attention to the areas where the cat spends most of his time. Inside the home spray every conceivable crack and crevice where ticks might hide, including baseboards, closets, clothing, furniture—everything.

Look for ticks throughout your cat's hair coat. Favorite hiding places are inside the ears and between the toes. Although a flea and tick shampoo is helpful, a dip is the most effective remedy available to remove ticks from your cat's body. If a female is dug into the skin and is in the process of engorging, it is important to remove it. First, put a drop or two of alcohol on the body. It will serve as an antiseptic and help loosen the grip. Using a tweezers, grasp the tick as close to the skin as possible. Twist the body in a counterclock direction as you pull it out. This will help prevent the head from breaking off and remaining in the skin. Always dispose of the ticks you remove by burning them or dropping them in a container of alcohol. Use an alcohol swab to clean the wound or dab it with an antibiotic ointment. Most pet supply stores and mail-order catalogs have available many effective products for treating your cat. Some veterinary clinics will dip the cat for you.

Mites. There are many varieties of mites, and they attack the cat's body in different ways. The *demodectic mange mite* is present at the base of the hair of most cats from birth. It is unknown why it causes disease in some cats and not at all in most. Other mites are the *sarcoptic mange mite* and the *ear mange mite*. Whenever your kitten or cat keeps pawing at her ears or if there is an apparent inflammation, you can assume it is the very common ear mite.

These are tiny, parasitic arachnids, barely visible to the naked eye, causing great discomfort and medical problems for cats. They are minuscule white creatures that can be seen moving if you look carefully and which cause the formation of a dark, crusty material in the ear canals of infected cats.

Demodectic mange is a serious parasitic skin disease. It involves hair loss around the head and front legs. The exposed skin becomes reddened and scaly. It is completely curable except for some advanced, untreated cases.

Sarcoptic mange is the cause of irritating itching, loss of hair, and crusting of the skin. The most affected areas are the ears, front legs, chest, and abdomen. It often leads to a bacterial skin infection that produces scabs over large portions of the body.

Demodectic and sarcoptic mange mites must be identified under a microscope. A scraping of skin is taken from the cat for this purpose. Treatment of all mites requires a veterinarian, whose instructions must be carried out faithfully.

FIRST AID FOR CATS

First aid for cats means emergency care until you can get veterinary help, and it can be your first line of defense in saving an animal's life. It is by no means a cure and should be followed up with an immediate visit to a veterinarian.

First Aid Kit

The first, most important step in maintaining the health of your cat is to be prepared for emergencies. It is advisable to develop a first aid kit that is conveniently located in your home. It should contain the following:

MEDICATIONS

Activated charcoal (for poisoning)
Antibacterial ointment
   For the eyes
   For the skin
Antiseptic powder or spray
Aromatic spirits of ammonia
Hydrogen peroxide (3% solution)
Ipecac (to induce vomiting)

Kaopectate
Milk of magnesia tablets (5gm)
Styptic powder (to stop minor bleeding)
Vaseline

MATERIALS AND PARAPHERNALIA

Absorbent cotton balls
Adhesive tape
Cotton applicators
Gauze bandage (1" and 2")
Gauze dressing pads (3" x 3")
Gauze pads (large and small)
Rectal thermometer
Scissors
Tongue depressors
Tweezers

It is now possible to find preassembled first aid kits at various pet supply outlets or in mail-order catalogs. However, the best ones are assembled at home by the cat owner.

Be prepared. Many communities have emergency veterinary services available twenty-four hours a day; ask your veterinarian or your local veterinary medical association about this. Learn whom to contact and keep the phone number handy. Read and learn the following first aid and emergency treatment procedures beforehand so you are familiar with the signs of conditions. Practice the techniques described so that you feel comfortable when administering first aid.

When Your Cat Is Hurt

Be careful when approaching an injured animal. An animal that is frightened or in pain may try to bite or scratch you, so protect yourself for the animal's safety—as well as your own.

Restraining your cat. A cat can be restrained by wrapping her in a blanket, towel, or coat. Then place the animal on her chest in a box to keep her quiet. Never force a cat into a position it does not want to be in. If you *are* bitten by a sick or injured cat, contact your physician as soon as possible.

Transporting an injured cat. An injured animal will assume the least painful position by himself, so do not change his position any more than necessary. Any animal that cannot stand should be carried on a stretcher made from a board or other flat object. Slide the stretcher carefully under the animal or grasp the loose skin along his backbone to pull him onto the stretcher. If it seems best to secure the animal, do not strap him so tightly that you interfere with his breathing—you could aggravate internal injuries as well. If no board is available, two or more people can transport an injured cat on a blanket lifted as flatly as possible by the four corners.

If you must move an animal by yourself, lift him with as little movement of the spine as possible. Place one arm under the rump and hind legs. Try to prevent the middle from sagging. With your other hand, try to keep the neck and head from flopping. Move slowly and carefully—rough handling or transport may worsen an animal's condition and increase the risk of shock.

Bite wound. Signs: open wounds, punctures, hair loss, salivating, pus or blood matted in the hair, sore swellings, elevated temperature.

Treatment: Clip the hair from around the wound, taking care not to cut the skin, then clean the wound with mild soap and warm water. Apply a bandage only to stop bleeding. Most bite wounds will become infected without professional treatment and may form an abscess, which can be a serious complication. Bites may cause internal damage that is not readily visible. For severe abdominal wounds, apply a wide bandage to hold the internal organs in, if necessary; lightly wrap the trunk from the shoulders to the pelvis.

Heatstroke. Any overheated cat can suffer from heatstroke. The most susceptible cats are those that are fat, aging, have chronic heart or lung disease, or those with "peke-faces" such as Persians. It is best to do what is necessary to avoid this life-threatening condition.

Never leave a cat in a car in warm, humid weather, even with the windows open. Never confine your pet in a small, poorly ventilated cat carrier on a hot, humid day, especially in a car, whether it is moving or not. Animals prone to heatstroke should be exercised only during the cool part of the day in warm weather. All animals need free access to shade and cool water in warm weather.

Signs: rapid breathing, loud panting, weakness, staggering, collapse, or unconsciousness, usually brought on by overexposure to the sun, overexercising in hot weather, or being left in a hot car.

Treatment: place the cat in a cool, shady spot with fresh air. Reduce body temperature by gently hosing the animal or soaking him in a partially filled tub of cool water. Use a rectal thermometer to monitor the animal's temperature; do not allow it to go below 103°F. If these measures do not bring immediate improvement, take the animal to a veterinarian without delay.

Bleeding. External bleeding is apparent. It comes from wounds. It requires control of blood loss and prevention of infection. Superficial wounds show slight blood loss. Wash with soap and water and apply an antiseptic. Smear on a light film of Vaseline and cover with a gauze pad and tape. For persistent bleeding, it may be necessary to use a pressure bandage. For this, apply a gauze bandage or cloth strips bound tightly around several times in order to create pressure over the bleeding cat. Cover the bandage completely with adhesive tape. If no tape is available, tie the gauze or cloth strip by tearing it down the center and knotting the two ends.

Severe or deep cuts are serious. A severed artery shows light-colored blood rushing quickly. Dark-colored blood that flows slowly is from a vein. These types of lacerations or punctures extend beyond the skin into the tissue beneath. Place a gauze pad over the wound and apply pressure with your hand for several minutes, allowing the blood to collect on the dressing and clot. If the blood soaks through, keep applying one pad on top of another. Maintain pressure on the wound.

Wrap completely with bandaging and cover the entire bandage with tape. See a veterinarian immediately.

Shock. A state of shock may be caused by severe fright, injury, or internal bleeding. It is a state of collapse caused by a failure of peripheral circulation. Look for apathy, prostration, weak pulse, hyperventilation, thirst, pale gums and eyelids, low body temperature or lower, cool extremities, and panting. To prevent shock, bleeding must be arrested, pain relieved, and infection prevented. Reassure the animal, talking quietly as you might to a frightened child, and help preserve the cat's body heat with a blanket (no electrical appliances). Keep the animal quiet and rush him to a veterinarian.

Shock, unfortunately, is often difficult to recognize because it may not appear until after an accident, as much as eight to ten hours later, when the cat is no longer being watched closely.

A cat in shock will frequently be thirsty, but giving it water could be dangerous. In severe shock, the digestive track will not efficiently absorb water. A semiconscious cat may accidentally inhale rather than swallow water. The most effective way of increasing blood volume is by intravenous transfusion, which must be administered by a veterinarian.

Broken bones. Bone fractures can be determined by loss of ability to bear body weight, deformity, abnormal angulation, swelling in the affected area, or protrusion of bone through the skin. A *simple fracture* is one break. A *comminuted fracture* involves two or more breaks. A *compound fracture* is a break that has punctured its surrounding tissue and may even protrude from the skin.

Restrain the cat immediately and as gently as possible. Immobilize the injured area with a splint. Use any firm object, such as a small plank of wood, a tree branch, heavy cardboard, even a metal tool, so long as it is long enough to brace the area above and below the break. Use gauze or cloth strips to wrap the limb or other broken area in a layer of absorbent cotton or newspaper so that the splint will be padded evenly. Fix the splint with bandage, rope, twine, or whatever you can find. Do not tie it too tightly. *Do not attempt to set the bone yourself.* Treat the animal for shock and rush him to the veterinarian.

Burns. Burns are caused either by direct flame, electricity, friction, corrosive chemicals, or scalding from hot liquids. The most common burns come from scalding water or other kitchen-related items such as soup, stew, or coffee.

The most important remedy for first- or second-degree burns (where skin has *not* been destroyed) is to lower the temperature of the burned area with cold water or cold towels soaked in ice water. The sooner the area is cooled, the less tissue is damaged. Apply a thick film of antibiotic ointment, such as Bacitracin, and bandage with a covering of gauze pads and rolled gauze. *Do not use home remedies such as butter, lard, and so on.* Look for signs of shock, breathing difficulties, or coughing and see the veterinarian immediately.

For deep burns or burns of more than 50 percent of the body, apply bandage or cloth soaked in cold water and seek immediate veterinary care.

Poison. Poisoning is a large, complex subject, too complex for the limitations of this text. Find the telephone number of the nearest poison control center in your area and keep it handy. Signs of poisoning are stomach pains and maybe howling, whimpering or yelping, vomiting, convulsions, muscle tremors, and labored breathing. Try to determine the source of the poison, but seek immediate help from the poison control center and your veterinarian. If possible, be prepared to tell them what you suspect the poisoning agent is. The empty container or jar that held the offending substance should be at hand to tell them the brand name, lot number, date, and list of ingredients. The label may also suggest antidotes and/or warn against certain types of treatment.

PART TWO

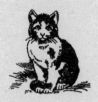

The Breeds

Based on The Show Standards of the Cat Fanciers' Association, Inc.

BREEDS ACCEPTED FOR REGISTRATION
BY THE CAT FANCIERS' ASSOCIATION, INC.

Longhair

American Curl (Longhair)
Balinese
Birman
Cymric
Javanese

Maine Coon Cat
Norwegian Forest Cat
Persian
Somali
Turkish Angora

Shorthair

Abyssinian
American Curl (Shorthair)
American Shorthair
American Wirehair
Bombay
British Shorthair
Burmese
Chartreux
Colorpoint Shorthair
Cornish Rex
Devon Rex
Egyptian Mau

Exotic Shorthair
Havana Brown
Japanese Bobtail
Korat
Manx
Ocicat
Oriental Shorthair
Russian Blue
Scottish Fold
Siamese
Singapura
Tonkinese

OTHER THAN CFA BREEDS

No Standards Given

Longhair

Himalayan
Kashmir

Ragdoll
Turkish Van

Shorthair

Bengal
California Spangled

Snowshoe
Sphynx

PET OWNERS—CAT FANCIERS

Which are the best cats? Are they the ones with the powder-puff coats, that are blown dry and born to win in cat shows? Or are they the ones with splotches and stripes that rule the homes of the everyday cat lover? Some people think of the best as Morris, Sylvestor, Toonsis, and Garfield blended together as one fantastic king of the carpet. Perfection, it would seem, is in the eye of the beholder.

Actually, it is a cat's personality and behavior that should be the primary source of a pet owner's appreciation for his or her home companion. A cat's unique way of relating to you and the rest of the world is what makes her so endearing. However, when considering cat ownership, one cannot ignore the distinction between *pet owners* and *cat fanciers*. Although they very often cross lines, these two groups are involved with *felis domesticus* in different ways.

Pet owners regard their cats as members of the family and expect them to give love, companionship, and unqualified acceptance in exchange for good food and a warm place to sleep. It is a fair deal. A pet cat is a four-legged love object enjoying the status of a rich relative. Her faults are regarded as endearing qualities and are almost always forgiven.

Cat fanciers are most often serious breeders and exhibitors of pure-breed cats. They could be considered practical historians and archivists of the breed or breeds with which they are involved. They are in a daily struggle to preserve (and improve if they can) the very best qualities of pure-breed cats. The aesthetic beauty and unique breed temperament of any given cat breed can only be continued if someone understands and practices the science of genetics and animal husbandry.

PURE-BREED CATS

Those who prefer pure-breed cats are either attracted to the look and the personality of a breed as a pet or have an interest in showing cats. According to CFA literature, "Cat breeds can be divided into three types: *natural, man-made,* and *spontaneous mutation. Natural breeds* such as the Persian, Russian Blue, Turkish Angora, and others were formed in nature's crucible, then sylized by cat fanciers through selective breeding. *Man-made* breeds—the Exotic Shorthair and Bombay, to name a few examples—were created by cat lovers who artfully combined existing breeds. *Spontaneous mutations* like the Manx and Scottish Fold are the consequence of nature's whimsical scrambling of the genetic code, which results in the taillessness in the Manx and the demurely capped ears in the Fold that are the respective signatures of these breeds."

Pure-breed cats are selected for mating because of their best characteristics and removed from breeding programs because of their faulty characteristics. All characteristics are measured against a written standard for each individual breed and put forth by national breed clubs and national registry organizations. Temperamentally defective, physically impaired, or otherwise seriously flawed examples of a breed are not usually mated by serious cat breeders.

There is a broad range of physical and mental differences among the cat breeds, and they are quite pronounced. One need only observe the Persian next to the Siamese to see the contrast in appearance and temperament. Among serious breeders and exhibitors in the Cat Fancy, the primary goal is to develop, improve, and preserve the various established breeds and their standards.

To the cat breeder a pure-breed cat comes from a line of traceable descendants of mutual ancestry. Such cats possess genetically governed variants, consistently producing similar traits and characteristics in their offspring as a result of a controlled breeding program. The offspring of pure-breed cats must be registered with a cat association if they are to authenticate their pure-breed status.

MIXED-BREED CATS

The majority of pet cats are mixed-breeds. They are the result of random matings of various cat breeds or from other mixed-breed cats. They almost never resemble the standard of any cat breed. They are usually not registered, have no pedigree (record of ancestors), and are not considered pure-breeds. Owners of such cats have no interest in these matters. In the United States these animals may be referred to as *house cats* or *alley cats*. In Great Britain they are sometimes called *moggs*. However, the Cat Fancy has gone to great lengths to acknowledge the desirability of *all* cats by allowing household pets to be registered (by some cat associations) and by encouraging a household pet competition for ribbons and prizes in most cat shows. To qualify for entry household pets must be altered (except for kittens), have all of their physical properties (except for a tail in the case of Manx types), and may not be declawed. Unlike pure-breeds, they are not judged according to a written standard but on the basis of physical condition, cleanliness, presentation, temperament, and attractive or unusual appearance. Throughout the world, cats of unknown lineage comprise the vast majority of house pets, and most of them are mixed-breeds. They are, without a doubt, the most popular cats of all.

NATIONAL CAT ASSOCIATIONS

When pure-breed kittens are born, the litter is usually registered with a national cat registering association such as the CFA (Cat Fanciers' Association, Inc.) or any one of the five American and one Canadian associations. Each individual kitten is later registered by its owner so that individual registration papers can be issued along with a complete pedigree (family history). This allows the registry to maintain complete records of all pure-breed cats.

The registration papers and pedigree are proof of a breeder's claims about a cat's breed, family history, and winning status at cat shows. These are the provable facts that qualify all pure-breed cats for showing and breeding according to the rules of the various cat associations, so long as it is a breed recognized by the association of choice. No breeder who shows cats will use a non-pedigreed, unregistered cat in a breeding program. They are not allowed to enter such cats in championship competition or register their offspring. Regulating cat shows (and those who judge them) and establishing who wins at them is another of the major functions of a national cat association.

The interest in pure-breed cats grow larger each year, with a constantly expanding Cat Fancy. In the United States and Canada there are six organizations that register pure-breed cats, maintain pedigrees, create and support breed standards, and sanction cat shows and the judges who preside over them. These organizations include the American Cat Association (ACA); the American Cat Fanciers' Association (ACFA); the Canadian Cat Association (CCA); the Cat Fanciers' Association (CFA); the Cat Fanciers' Federation (CFF); and The International Cat Association (TICA).

The largest cat registry in the world is the Cat Fanciers' Association, Inc. (CFA), with close to six hundred affiliate clubs in the United States, Canada, and Japan. It generates over three hundred cat shows a year, which attract a total of almost seventy thousand entries. The American Cat Association is the oldest organization in the United States and registers pure-breed cats with over forty member clubs. The International Cat Association (TICA) is a relatively new organization with growing influence in the United States, offering the established cat associations their greatest challenge ever. Still, CFA is considered to be the feline counterpart to the American Kennel Club in terms of size and prestige.

For pure-breed enthusiasts the choice of associations is large and varied. However, it is important to understand that no two cat associations accept or register all of the breeds available. For example, CFA, at this writing, registers thirty-three breeds.

But there are at least forty breeds accepted by one or more of the six cat associations. Each breed is allowed a specific variety of coat colors and patterns in its official standard, which means that there may be dozens of different-looking cats of the same breed. For example, the Persian comes in fifty-six coat colors and color combinations approved by the Cat Fanciers' Association. In contrast, the association allows the Bombay to be shown in solid black only. The Himalayan is considered to be a separate breed by most cat associations, except the CFA, which considers it to be a color-pointed variety of the Persian. These differences are outlined by every cat association in a set of *breed standards*. A breed standard is a precise, written description of a breed. The standard, according to CFA literature, "is an abstract aesthetic ideal."

For those who want to know more about pure-breed cats, for the purpose of acquiring one or for grasping what the goals are at a cat show, we present the Show Standards of the Cat Fanciers' Association, Inc. These are the written standards for every breed that is accepted for registration and/or showing by the CFA. Here are the aesthetic ideals for which everyone who shows their cats is working. The Author's Note preceding each breed's standard is a subjective statement that is *not* part of the official standards. It is simply meant to offer a bit of additional information not included in the standards. A glossary of terms follows the CFA Standards, which should prove to be useful to those not familiar with the terminology of the cat show world.

It is important to understand that the CFA Show Standards change every year to a slight degree. New breeds are occasionally added. It is impossible to remain completely current. However, even though the standards change slightly from year to year, the essential features of each breed remain constant. It is hoped that these CFA Show Standards will help all cat-loving enthusiasts.

THE SHOW STANDARDS OF THE CAT FANCIERS' ASSOCIATION, INC.

ABYSSINIAN

AUTHOR'S NOTE—Abyssinians are the motorcycles of the cat breeds, with their fast starts and speedy runs around the house. They are highly spirited, affectionate, and extremely playful cats. They came from Abyssinia (Ethiopia) or Egypt three or four thousand years ago. They may have descended from two small African wild cat species. Some have written that they are descended from the ancient caffre cats or the sacred cats of Egypt. An Aby was probably the first cat in history to appear in a painting, in an Egyptian tomb about four thousand years ago. Abyssinians first arrived in North America around the turn of the twentieth century.

CFA Show Standards

POINT SCORE

HEAD (25)
    Muzzle 6
    Skull 6
    Ears 7
    Eye Shape 6
BODY (30)
    Torso 15
    Legs and Feet 10
    Tail 5
COAT (10)
    Texture 10
COLOR (35)
    Color 15
    Ticking 15
    Eye Color 5

GENERAL: The overall impression of the ideal Abyssinian would be a colorful cat with a distinctly ticked coat, medium in size, and regal in appearance. The Abyssinian is lithe, hard, and muscular, showing eager activity and a lively interest in all surroundings. Well balanced temperamentally and physically with all elements of the cat in proportion.

HEAD: A modified, slightly rounded wedge without flat planes, the brow, cheek, and profile lines all showing a gentle contour. A slight rise from the bridge of the nose to the forehead, which should be of good size, with width between the ears and flowing into the arched neck without a break.

MUZZLE: Not sharply pointed or square. The chin should be neither receding nor protruding. Allowance should be made for jowls in adult males.

EARS: Alert, large, and moderately pointed; broad, cupped at the base, and set as though listening. Hair on ears very short and close-lying, preferably tipped with black or dark brown on a ruddy Abyssinian, chocolate brown on a red Abyssinian, slate blue on the blue Abyssinian, and light cocoa brown on the fawn Abyssinian.

EYES: Almond-shaped, large, brilliant, and expressive. Neither round nor oriental. Eyes accentuated by fine dark line, encircled by light colored area.

BODY: Medium long, lithe, and graceful, but showing well-developed muscular strength without coarseness. Abyssinian conformation strikes a medium between the extremes of the cobby and the svelte lengthy type. Proportion and general balance more to be desired than mere size.

LEGS and FEET: Proportionately slim, fine-boned. The Abyssinian stands well off the ground, giving the impression of being on tiptoe. Paws small, oval, and compact. Toes: five in front and four behind.

TAIL: Thick at base, fairly long and tapering.

COAT: Soft, silky, fine in texture, but dense and resilient to the touch, with a lustrous sheen. Medium in length but long enough to accommodate two or three dark bands of ticking.

PENALIZE: Off-color pads. Long, narrow head; short, round head. Barring on legs; dark, broken necklace markings; rings on tail. Coldness or gray tones in the coat.

DISQUALIFY: White locket, or white anywhere other than nostril, chin, and upper throat area. Kinked or abnormal tail. Dark, unbroken necklace. Gray undercoat close to the skin extending throughout a major portion of the body. Any black hair on red Abyssinian. Incorrect number of toes.

ABYSSINIAN COLORS

Ruddy, red, blue, and fawn.

Coat color: Warm and glowing. **Ticking:** Distinct and even, with dark-colored bands contrasting with lighter-colored bands on the hair shafts. Undercoat color clear and bright to the skin. Deeper color shades desired, however intensity of ticking not to be sacrificed for depth of color. Darker shading along spine allowed if fully ticked. Preference given to cats UNMARKED on the undersides, chest, and legs; tail without rings. **Facial markings:** Dark lines extending from eyes and brows, cheekbone shading, dots and shading on whisker pads are all desirable enhancements. Eyes accentuated by fine dark line, encircled by light-colored area. **Eye color:** Gold or green, the more richness and depth of color the better.

Abyssinian allowable outcross breeds: None.

AMERICAN CURL

AUTHOR'S NOTE: The American Curl is one of the most recent breeds to be accepted by the CFA for registration and showing. This unusual breed was first reported as a spontaneous mutation by Joe and Grace Ruga of Lakewood, California, owners of the foundation cat, Shulamith, from which all pedigreed American Curls descend. The distinctive feature of the breed is the unusual formation of the ears. On this breed the ears are firm to the touch, erect, and open, curving up in a gentle curl. American Curls are being developed with longhair and shorthair coats.

CFA Show Standards
(Provisional Standard)

POINT SCORE

HEAD (15)
 Profile 6
 Shape 6
 Size 3
EARS (25)
 Degree of Curl 8
 Shape 7
 Size 6
 Placement 3
 Furnishings 1
EYES (10)
 Shape 3
 Size 3
 Placement 3
 Color 1
BODY (35)
 Shape 7
 Size and Boning 7
 Tail 5
 Legs and Feet 5
 Balance and Condition 5
 Musculature 4
 Neck 2
COAT AND COLOR (15)
 Texture 7
 Length 6
 Color 2

GENERAL: The American Curl occurred as a spontaneous mutation in Southern California. All bona fide American Curls are descended from Shulamith, the foundation female.

The distinctive feature of the breed is their unique, attractively curled ears, set on the corners of the head, with the base of the ears firm and tips soft and flexible. Erect and open, curving in a smooth arc back away from the face, they point toward the center of the base of the skull.

The American Curl is a well-balanced, intermediately sized cat, weighing five to ten pounds and taking two to three years to reach maturity. Allowance is made for normal male characteristics.

HEAD: **Profile**—Nose straight, slight rise from bottom of eyes to forehead, gentle curve to top of skull, chin firm. **Shape**—Modified wedge, muzzle break, gently contoured. **Muzzle**—Neither pointed nor square, gentle transition. **Size**—Intermediate.

EARS: **Shape**—Wide at base, curving back in a smooth arc, rounded tips. **Degree of curl**—90-degree arc or better but not to exceed 180; most continuous curl desired. **Size**—Moderately large. **Placement**—Erect, set on corners of head, facing outward at a slight angle, curling back away from the face, toward the center of the base of the skull. **Furnishings**—Interior furnishings well extended, tufts desirable.

EYES: **Shape**—Walnut. **Size**—Moderately large. **Placement**—Centered on face between base of ear and tip of nose; on a slight bias, one eye width apart. **Color**—No relationship to coat color, except blue eyes in pointed divisions.

BODY: **Shape**—Semi-foreign, length 1½ times the height at the shoulder. **Size and boning**—Intermediate, neither heavy nor fine. **Tail**—Wide at base, tapering, in proportion to body length at shoulder. **Legs and feet**—Intermediate, neither heavy nor fine, straight when viewed from front or rear. Feet medium and round. **Musculature**—Moderately developed strength and tone. **Neck**—In proportion to head and body.

COAT and COLOR (LONGHAIR): **Texture**—Silky, minimal undercoat. **Length**—Semi-long, lying flat, tail coat full and plumed.

COAT and COLOR (SHORTHAIR): **Texture**—Soft, minimal undercoat. **Length**—Short, lying flat, not close-lying. Tail coat same length as body coat.

PENALIZE: **Ears**—Low set, mismatched, donkey ears; abrupt change of direction without a smooth arc as in pinched, vertical crimp, horizontal kink, thickened or calcified ears, and ears where interior surface appears to be corrugated. **Nose**— Deep nose break. **Coat**—Heavy undercoat, ruffs, coarse texture. **Color**—Buttons, lockets.

WITHHOLD WINS: Tail faults.

DISQUALIFY: An extreme curl—In an adult cat, where the tip of the ear touches the back of the ear or the head. Any ear lacking firm cartilage from the base to at least a third of its height. Any cat with straight ears.

AMERICAN CURL COLORS

White, black, blue, red, cream, chocolate, lilac, chinchilla silver, shaded silver, chinchilla golden, shaded golden, shell cameo, shaded cameo, shell tortoiseshell, shaded tortoiseshell, black smoke, blue smoke, cameo smoke, chocolate smoke, lavender smoke, cream smoke, smoke tortoiseshell, chocolate tortoiseshell smoke, blue-cream smoke, classic tabby pattern, mackerel tabby pattern, patched tabby, spotted tabby pattern, ticked tabby pattern, brown patched tabby, blue patched tabby, silver patched tabby, silver tabby, red tabby, brown tabby, blue tabby, cream tabby, blue silver and cream silver tabbies, chocolate silver tabby, lavender silver tabby, cameo tabby, tortoiseshell, calico, diluted calico, blue-cream, bi-color, van bi-color, van calico, van dilute calico, tabby and white, seal point, chocolate point, blue point, lilac point, lilac-lynx point, lilac-cream point, lilac-cream lynx point, flame (red) point, cream point, cream lynx point, tortie point, chocolate-tortie point, chocolate-tortie lynx point, blue-cream point, chocolate lynx point, seal lynx point, blue lynx point, tortie-lynx point, and blue-cream lynx point.

OACC (Other American Curl Colors): All accepted pointed colors with white. Any other color or pattern.

American Curl allowable outcross breeds: None.

AMERICAN SHORTHAIR

AUTHOR'S NOTE: Although this breed is descended from the basic European working cat, it is considered one of the few truly American cat breeds. The American Shorthair is considered by many to be a "working cat" because of its great hunting skills. It is often confused with the basic, nonpedigreed cat that it seems to resemble. The difference between the common house cat and the uncommon American Shorthair is tremendous. Since 1904 skilled cat people have with great success been selectively breeding the best specimens for their physical and mental excellence. The American Shorthair differs from all common cats in that it has been bred for many generations to meet breed standards that keep it strong, muscular, intelligent, and lively. It is athletic, sweet-natured, independent, and highly dignified.

CFA Show Standard

POINT SCORE

Head (including size and shape of eyes, ear shape, and set and structure of nose.) 30
Type (including shape, size, bone, and length of tail.) . . 25
Coat 15
Color 20
(Tabby pattern = 10 points; Color = 10 points)
Eye color 10

GENERAL: The American Shorthair is a true breed of working cat. The conformation should be adapted for this, with no part of the anatomy so exaggerated as to foster weakness. The general effect should be that of a strongly built, well-balanced, symmetrical cat with conformation indicating power, endurance, and agility.

SIZE: Medium to large. No sacrifice of quality for sake of size. Females may be less massive in all respects than males.

PROPORTIONS: Slightly longer than tall. (Height is profile measure from top of shoulder blades to ground. Length is profile measure from tip of breastbone to rear tip of buttocks.) Viewed from side, body can be divided into three equal parts: from tip of breastbone to elbow, from elbow to front of hind leg, and from front of hind leg to rear tip of buttocks. Length of tail is equal to distance from shoulder blades to base of tail.

HEAD: Large, with full-cheeked face giving the impression of an oblong just slightly longer than wide. Sweet, open expression. Viewed from front, head can be divided in two equal parts: from base to ears to middle of eyes and from middle of eyes to chin tip.

EARS: Medium size, slightly rounded at tips and not unduly open at base. Distance between ears, measured from lower inner corners, twice distance between eyes.

FOREHEAD: Viewed in profile, forehead forms smooth, moderately convex, continuous curve flowing over top of head into neck. Viewed from front, there is no dome between ears.

EYES: Large and wide with upper lid shaped like half an almond (cut lengthwise) and lower lid shaped in a fully rounded curve. At least width of one eye between eyes. Outer corners set very slightly higher than inner corners. Bright, clear, and alert. *[Depending on the coat color, eye color should be either brilliant gold, deep blue, green or blue-green, hazel, or brilliant copper.]*

NOSE: Medium length, same width for entire length. Viewed in profile, gentle, concavely curved rise from bridge of nose to forehead.

MUZZLE: Squared. Definite jowls in mature males.

JAWS: Strong and long enough to successfully grasp prey. Both level and scissors bites considered equally correct. (In level bite, top and bottom front teeth meet evenly. In scissors bite, inside edge of top front teeth touch outside edge of lower front teeth.)

CHIN: Firm and well-developed, forming perpendicular line with upper lip.

NECK: Medium in length, muscular, and strong.

BODY: Solidly built, powerful, and muscular with well-developed shoulders, chest, and hindquarters. Back broad, straight, and level. Viewed in profile, slight slope down from hip bone to base of tail. Viewed from above, outer lines of body parallel.

LEGS: Medium in length and bone, heavily muscled. Viewed from rear, all four legs straight and parallel, with paws facing forward.

PAWS: Firm, full, and rounded, with heavy pads. Toes: five in front, four behind.

TAIL: Medium long, heavy at base, tapering to abrupt blunt end in appearance but with normal tapering final vertebrae.

COAT: Short, thick, even, and hard in texture. Regional and seasonal variation in coat thickness allowed. Coat dense enough to protect from moisture, cold, and superficial skin injuries.

PENALIZE: Excessive cobbiness or ranginess. Very short tail.

DISQUALIFY: Any appearance of hybridization with any other breed, including long or fluffy fur, deep nose break, bulging eye set, brow ridge. Kinked or abnormal tail. Locket or button (white spots on colors not specifying same). Incorrect number of toes. Undershot or overshot bite. Obesity or emaciation. Any feature so exaggerated as to foster weakness.

AMERICAN SHORTHAIR COLORS

White, black, blue, red, cream, chinchilla silver, shaded silver, shell cameo (red chinchilla), shaded cameo (red shaded), black smoke, blue smoke, cameo smoke (red smoke), tortoiseshell smoke, classic tabby pattern, mackerel tabby pattern, patched tabby pattern, brown patched tabby, blue patched tabby, silver patched tabby, silver tabby (classic, mackerel), red tabby (classic, mackerel), brown tabby (classic, mackerel), blue tabby (classic, mackerel), cream tabby (classic, mackerel), cameo tabby (classic, mackerel), tortoiseshell, calico, dilute calico, blue-cream, bi-color, van bi-color, van calico, van blue-cream and white.

American Shorthair allowable outcross breeds: None.

AMERICAN WIREHAIR

AUTHOR'S NOTE: The American Wirehair's origins can be traced to one cat, "Council Rock Farm Adam of Hi-Fi." He and his sister "Tip-Toe" were born with fur more like sheep wool than the traditional coats of their common cat parents. The breed is now considered a mutation of the American Shorthair. Since its first appearance, it has been bred to type with the American Shorthair as its necessary outcross and has become an original American cat breed. These cats are more reserved than their American Shorthair cousins but grow into loving, unassuming pets with pleasing personalities.

CFA Show Standard

POINT SCORE

Head (including size and shape of eyes, ear shape and
 set.) 25
Type (including shape, size, bone and length of tail.) . . 20
Coat 45
Color and eye color 10

GENERAL: The American Wirehair is a spontaneous mutation. The coat, which is not only springy, dense, and resilient, but also coarse and hard to the touch, distinguishes the American Wirehair from all other breeds. Characteristic is activity, agility, and keen interest in its surroundings.

HEAD: In proportion to the body. Underlying bone structure is round, with prominent cheekbones and well-developed muzzle and chin. There is a slight whisker break.

NOSE: In profile the nose shows a gentle concave curve.

MUZZLE: Well-developed. Allowance for jowls in adult males.

CHIN: Firm and well-developed, with no apparent malocclusion.

EARS: Medium, slightly rounded at tips, set wide and not unduly open at the base.

EYES: Large, round, bright, and clear. Set well apart. Aperture has light upward tilt. *[Depending on the color, eye color should be deep blue, brilliant gold, green or blue-green, or hazel.]*

BODY: Medium to large. Back level, shoulders and hips same width, torso well-rounded and in proportion. Males larger than females.

LEGS: Medium in length and bone, well-muscled and proportionate to body.

PAWS: Oval and compact. Toes, five in front and four behind.

TAIL: In proportion to body, tapering from the well-rounded rump to a rounded tip, neither blunt nor pointed.

COAT: Springy, tight, medium in length. Individual hairs are crimped, hooked, or bent, including hair within the ears. The overall appearance of wiring and the coarseness and resilience of the coat are more important than the crimping of each hair. The density of the wired coat leads to ringlet formation rather than waves. That coat, which is very dense, resilient, crimped, and coarse, is most desirable, as are curly whiskers.

PENALIZE: Deep nose break. Long or fluffy fur.

DISQUALIFY: Incorrect coat. Kinked or abnormal tail. Incorrect number of toes. Evidence of hybridization resulting in the colors chocolate, lavender, the Himalayan pattern, or these combinations with white.

AMERICAN WIREHAIR COLORS

White, black, blue, red, cream, chinchilla silver, shaded silver, shell cameo (red chinchilla), shaded cameo (red shaded), black smoke, blue smoke, cameo smoke (red smoke), classic tabby pattern, mackerel tabby pattern, silver tabby (classic, mackerel), red tabby (classic, mackerel), brown tabby (classic, mackerel) blue tabby (classic, mackerel), cream tabby (classic, mackerel), cameo tabby (classic, mackerel), tortoiseshell, calico, dilute calico, blue-cream, and bi-color.

OWC (Other Wirehair Colors): Any other color or pattern with the exception of those showing evidence of hybridization resulting in the colors chocolate, lavender, the Himalayan pattern, or these combinations with white. **EYE COLOR**: Appropriate to the color of the cat.

American Wirehair allowable outcross breeds: American Shorthair.

BALINESE

AUTHOR'S NOTE: In the early 1960s Balinese cats were considered to be mutated Siamese cats with long hair. That view is no longer accepted. The Balinese is now recognized as a separate breed and is produced consistently by knowledge-able breeders. Named after the graceful dancers from Bali, these cats are allowed by CFA in the four traditional "point" colors of Siamese cats. See Javanese for more information. Their personalities are similar to those of all Siamese cats. They are very vocal and demanding of human attention. These are good-natured cats with an unquenchable curiosity. They insist on participating in all human activities.

CFA Show Standards

POINT SCORE

HEAD (20)
Long, flat profile 6
Wedge, fine muzzle, size 5
Ears 4
Chin 3
Width between eyes 2
EYES (5)
Shape, size, slant, and placement 5
BODY (30)
Structure and size, including neck 12
Muscle tone 10
Legs and Feet 5
Tail 3
COAT (20)
Length 10
Texture 10
COLOR (25)
Body color 10

Point color (matching points of dense color, proper
  foot pads and nose leather.) 10
Eye color 5

GENERAL: The ideal Balinese is a svelte cat with long, tapering lines, very lithe but strong and muscular. Excellent physical condition. Neither flabby nor bony. Not fat. Eyes clear. Because of the longer coat the Balinese appears to have softer lines and less extreme type than other breeds of cats with similar type.

HEAD: Long, tapering wedge. Medium size in good proportion to body. The total wedge starts at the nose and flares out in straight lines to the tips of the ears, forming a triangle, with no break at the whiskers. No less than the width of an eye between the eyes. When the whiskers and face hair are smoothed back, the underlying bone structure is apparent. Allowance must be made for jowls in the stud cat.

SKULL: Flat. In profile, a long, straight line should be felt from the top of the head to the tip of the nose. No bulge over the eyes. No dip in nose.

NOSE: Long and straight. A continuation of the forehead with no break.

MUZZLE: Fine, wedge-shaped.

CHIN and JAW: Medium size. Tip of chin lines up with tip of nose in the same vertical plane. Neither receding nor excessively massive.

EARS: Strikingly large, pointed, wide at base, continuing the lines of the wedge.

EYES: Almond-shaped. Medium size. Neither protruding nor recessed. Slanted toward the nose in harmony with lines of wedge and ears. Uncrossed.

BODY: Medium size. Graceful, long, and svelte. A distinctive combination of fine bones and firm muscles. Shoulders and hips continue same sleek lines of tubular body. Hips never wider than shoulders. Abdomen tight. The male may be somewhat larger than the female.

NECK: Long and slender.

LEGS: Bone structure long and slim. Hind legs higher than front. In good proportion to body.

PAWS: Dainty, small, and oval. Toes: five in front and four behind.

TAIL: Bone structure long, thin, tapering to a fine point. Tail hair spreads out like a plume.

COAT: Medium length, fine, silky without downy undercoat lying close to the body, the coat may appear shorter than it is. Hair is longest on the tail.

COLOR: **Body**—Even, with subtle shading when allowed. Allowance should be made for darker color in older cats, as Balinese generally darken with age, but there must be definite contrast between body color and points. **Points**—Mask, ears, legs, feet, tail dense and clearly defined. All of the same shade. Mask covers entire face including whisker pads and is connected to ears by tracings. Mask should not extend over top of head. No ticking or white hairs in points.

PENALIZE: Lack of pigment in the nose leather and/or paw pads in part or in total. Crossed eyes. Palpable and/or visible protrusion of the cartilage at the end of the sternum. Soft or mushy body.

DISQUALIFY: Any evidence of illness or poor health. Weak hind legs. Mouth breathing due to nasal obstruction or poor occlusion. Emaciation. Kink in tail. Eyes other than blue. White toes and/or feet. Incorrect number of toes. Definite double coat (i.e., downy undercoat).

BALINESE COLORS

BLUE POINT: Body bluish white, cold in tone, shading gradually to white on stomach and chest. Points deep blue. **Nose leather and Paw pads**—Slate-colored. **Eye color**—Deep vivid blue.

CHOCOLATE POINT: Body ivory with no shading. Points milk-chocolate color, warm in tone. **Nose leather and Paw pads**—Cinnamon-pink. **Eye color**—Deep vivid blue.

LILAC POINT: Body glacial white with no shading. Points frosty gray with pinkish tone. **Nose leather and Paw pads**—Lavender-pink. **Eye color**—Deep vivid blue.

SEAL POINT: Body even pale fawn to cream, warm in tone, shading gradually into lighter color on the stomach and chest. Points deep seal brown. **Nose leather and Paw pads**—Same color as points. **Eye color**—Deep vivid blue.

Balinese allowable outcross breeds: Siamese.

BIRMAN
(Sacred Cat of Burma)

AUTHOR'S NOTE: The Birman is a very playful, intelligent, and active cat. It is also a family-loving cat that has little or no tolerance for solitude. It thrives on the company of people, cats, and other pets. This beautiful breed comes to us from history and legend. These were the temple cats of Lao-Tsun and were much loved by the Buddhist priests. They have been called the Tibetan Temple Cats. Because two Europeans, August Pavie and Major Russell-Gordon, helped the priests escape Burma during a perilous time, they were given a pair of Birmans in 1919. The cats have been carefully nurtured in France since that time. They came to North America around 1960. The Birman is a unique, natural cat. It is not Siamese or Persian, although the color points and long coat could lead one to think so. The white gloves on all four paws are a positive identification. This charming, bright cat is more than an object of beauty.

CFA Show Standards

POINT SCORE

HEAD, BODY, TYPE and COAT (65)

Head (including boning, nose, jaw, chin, profile, ear and eye shape and set.) 30

Body/Type (including boning, stockiness, elongation, legs, tail.) 25

Coat (including length, texture, ruff.) 10

COLOR—INCLUDING EYE COLOR (35)

Color except gloves (including body color, point color, eye color.) 15

GENERAL: A cat of mystery and legend, the Birman is a color-pointed cat with long, silky hair and four pure white feet. It is strongly built, elongated, and stocky, neither svelte nor cobby. The distinctive head has strong jaws, a firm chin, a medium-length Roman nose with nostrils set low on the nose leather. There should be good width between the ears, which are medium in size. The blue, almost round eyes are set well apart, giving a sweet expression to the face.

HEAD: Skull strong, broad, and rounded. There is a slight flat spot just in front of the ears.

NOSE: Medium in length and width, in proportion to size of head. Roman shape in profile. Nostrils set low on the nose leather.

PROFILE: The forehead slopes back and is slightly convex. The medium-length nose, which starts just below the eyes, is Roman in shape (which is slightly convex), with the nostrils set low on the nose leather. The chin is strong, with the lower jaw forming a perpendicular line with the upper lip.

CHEEKS: Full, with somewhat rounded muzzle. The fur is short in appearance about the face, but to the extreme outer area of the cheek the fur is longer.

JAWS: Heavy.

CHIN: Strong and well-developed.

EARS: Medium in length. Almost as wide at the base as tall. Modified to a rounded point at the tip; set as much to the side as into the top of the head.

EYES: Almost round with a sweet expression. Set well apart, with the outer corner tilted VERY slightly upward. Blue in color, the deeper blue the better.

BODY: Long and stocky. Females may be proportionately smaller than males.

LEGS: Medium in length and heavy.

PAWS: Large, round, and firm. Five toes in front, four behind.

TAIL: Medium in length, in pleasing proportion to the body.

COAT: Medium long to long, silken in texture, with heavy ruff around the neck, slightly curly on stomach. This fur is of such a texture that it does not mat.

COLOR EXCEPT GLOVES: **Body**—Even, with subtle shading when allowed. Strong contrast between body color and points. **Points except gloves**—Mask, ears, legs, and tail dense and clearly defined, all of the same shade. Mask covers entire face, including whisker pads, and is connected to ears by tracings. No ticking or white hair in points. *Golden Mist*—Desirable in all point colors is the "golden mist," a faint golden beige cast on the back and sides. This is somewhat deeper in the seal points and may be absent in kittens.

GLOVES: **Front paws**—Have white gloves ending in an even line across the paw at, or between, the second or third joints. (The third joint is where the paw bends when the cat is standing.) The upper limit of white should be the metacarpal (dew) pad. (The metacarpal pad is the highest up little paw pad, located in the middle of the back of the front paw, above the third joint and just below the wrist bones.) Symmetry of the front gloves is desirable. **Back paws**—White glove covers all the toes, and may extend up somewhat higher than front gloves. Symmetry of the rear gloves is desirable. **Laces**—The gloves on the back paws must extend up the back of the hock and are called laces in this area. Ideally, the laces end in a point or inverted "V" and extend ½ to ¾ of the way up the hock. Lower or higher laces are acceptable, but should not go beyond the hock. Symmetry of the two laces is desirable. **Paw pads**—Pink preferred, but dark spot(s) on paw pad(s) acceptable because of the two colors in pattern. **Note**—Ideally, the front gloves match, the back gloves match, and the two laces match. Faultlessly gloved cats are a rare exception, and the Birman is to be judged on all its parts, as well as the gloves.

PENALIZE: White that does not run across the front paws in an even line. Persian- or Siamese-type head. Delicate bone structure. White shading on stomach and chest. Lack of laces on one or both back gloves. White beyond the metacarpal (dew) pad. (The metacarpal pad is the highest up little paw pad, located in the middle of the back of the front paw, above the third joint and just below the wrist bones.)

DISQUALIFY: Lack of white gloves on any paw. Kinked or abnormal tail. Crossed eyes. Incorrect number of toes. Areas of pure white in the points, if not connected to the gloves and part of or an extension of the gloves. Paw pads are part of the gloves. Areas of white connected to other areas of white by paw pads (of any color) are not cause for disqualification. Discrete areas of point color in the gloves, if not connected to point color of legs (exception, paw pads). White on back legs beyond the hock.

BIRMAN COLORS

SEAL POINT: Body even pale fawn to cream, warm in tone, shading gradually to lighter color on the stomach and chest. Points, except for gloves, deep seal brown. Gloves pure white. **Nose leather**—Same color as points. **Paw pads**—Pink. **Eye color**—Blue, the deeper and more violet the better.

BLUE POINT: Body bluish white to pale ivory, shading gradually to almost white on stomach and chest. Points, except for gloves, deep blue. Gloves pure white. **Nose leather**—Slate-color. **Paw pads**—Pink. **Eye color**—Blue, the deeper and more violet the better.

CHOCOLATE POINT: Body ivory with no shading. Points, except for gloves, milk-chocolate color, warm in tone. Gloves pure white. **Nose leather**—Cinnamon pink. **Paw pads**—Pink. **Eye color**—Blue, the deeper and more violet the better.

LILAC POINT: Almost white. Points, except for gloves, frosty gray with pinkish tone. Gloves pure white. **Nose leather**—Lavender-pink. **Paw pads**—Pink. **Eye color**—Blue, the deeper and more violet the better.

Birman allowable outcross breeds: None.

BOMBAY

AUTHOR'S NOTE: The Bombay is a quiet cat with a mild, easygoing manner. Most of these charming, graceful felines are good family cats and quite friendly, even with other cats. They are playful, soft-spoken, and very affectionate. The meeting of a Burmese and a black American Shorthair produced the first Bombay. This laconic lover was created in the 1950s in the United States, but it was named for the black leopards of India.

CFA Show Standards

POINT SCORE

HEAD AND EARS (25)
Roundness of head 7
Full face and proper profile 7
Ears 7
Chin 4
EYES (5)
Placement and shape 5
BODY (20)
Body 15
Tail 5
COAT (20)
Shortness 10
Texture 5
Close lying 5
COLOR (30)
Body color 20
Eye color 10

GENERAL: Due to its short, jet-black, gleaming coat and bright gold to vivid copper eyes, combined with a solid body and a sweet facial expression, the ideal Bombay has an unmistakable look of its own. It is a medium-size cat, well balanced, friendly, alert, and outgoing; muscular and having a surprising weight for its size. The body and tail should be of medium length, the head round with medium-sized, wide-set ears, a visible nose break, large, rounded, wide-set eyes, and be of excellent proportions and carriage.

HEAD: The head should be pleasingly rounded, with no sharp angles. The face should be full, with considerable breadth between the eyes, tapering slightly to a short, well-developed muzzle. In profile there should be a visible nose break; however, it should not present a "pugged" or "snubbed" look.

EARS: The ears should be medium in size and set well apart on a rounded skull, alert, tilting, slightly forward, broad at the base, and with slightly rounded tips.

CHIN: The chin should be firm, neither receding nor protruding, reflecting a proper bite.

EYES: Set far apart, with rounded aperture.

BODY: Medium in size, muscular in development, neither compact nor rangy. Allowance is to be made for larger size in males.

LEGS: In proportion to the body and tail.

PAWS: Round. Toes, five in front, four in back.

TAIL: Straight, medium in length; neither short nor "whippy."

COAT: Fine, short, satin-like texture; close-lying, with a shimmering patent-leather sheen.

PENALIZE: Excessive cobbiness or ranginess.

DISQUALIFY: Kinked or abnormal tail. Lockets or spots. Incorrect number of toes. Nose leather or paw pads other than black. Green eyes. Improper bite. Extreme break that interferes with normal breathing and tearing of eyes.

BOMBAY COLORS

COLOR: The mature specimen should be black to the roots. Kitten coats should darken and become more sleek with age. **Nose leather and paw pads**—Black. **Eye color**—Ranging from gold to copper, the greater the depth and brilliance the better.

BRITISH SHORTHAIR

AUTHOR'S NOTE: Considering its large size, the British Shorthair is an extremely placid, laid-back cat. Once kitten-

hood is over, its days of playfulness are left behind. It is a friendly cat, whose sense of dignity is sometimes mistaken for aloofness. The most pleasing aspect of the British Shorthair personality is its gentleness. The breed was created when the English began selectively breeding their pet cats in the nineteenth century. After World War I some Persian blood was added to create the plush, sophisticated cat we see today. The British Shorthair was accepted in the United States for registration and showing in the 1970s.

CFA Show Standards

POINT SCORE

HEAD (25)

    Muzzle and Chin 5

    Skull 5

    Ears 5

    Neck 5

    Eye Shape 5

BODY (35)

    Torso 20

    Legs and Paws 10

    Tail 5

COAT (20)

    Texture, length, and density 20

COLOR (20)

    Eye color 5

    Coat color 15

GENERAL: The British Shorthair is compact, well-balanced, and powerful, showing good depth of body, a full broad chest, short to medium strong legs, rounded paws, tail thick at base with a rounded tip. The head is round with good width between the ears, round cheeks, firm chin, medium ears, large, round, and well-opened eyes, and a medium broad nose. The coat is short and very dense. Females are less massive in all respects, with males having larger jowls. This breed is slow to mature.

HEAD: Round and massive. Round face, with round underlying bone structure well set on a short, thick neck. The forehead should be rounded, with a slight flat plane on the top of the head. The forehead should not slope.

NOSE: Medium, broad. In profile there is a gentle dip.

CHIN: Firm and well-developed.

MUZZLE: Distinctive, well-developed, with a definite stop beyond large, round whisker pads.

EARS: Ear set is important. Medium in size, broad at the base, rounded at the tips. Set far apart, fitting into (without distorting) the rounded contour of the head.

EYES: Large, round, well opened. Set wide apart and level. *[Depending upon coat color, eye color deep sapphire blue, gold, copper, green, or hazel.]*

BODY: Medium to large, well knit, and powerful. Level back and a deep, broad chest.

LEGS: Short to medium, well-boned, and strong. In proportion to the body. Forelegs are straight.

PAWS: Round and firm. Toes: five in front and four behind.

TAIL: Medium length in proportion to the body, thicker at base, tapering slightly to a rounded tip.

COAT: Short, very dense, well bodied, resilient and firm to the touch. Not double coated or woolly.

COLOR: For cats with special markings: 10 points for color and 10 points for markings. Shadow tabby markings in solid color, smoke, or bi-color kittens are not a fault.

PENALIZE: Definite nose stop. Overlong or light undercoat. Soft coat. Rangy body. Weak chin.*

DISQUALIFY: Incorrect eye color, green rims in adults. Tail defects. Long or fluffy coat. Incorrect number of toes. Locket or button. Improper color or pigment in nose leather and/or paw pads in part or total. Any evidence of illness or poor health. Any evidence of wryness of jaw, poor dentition (arrangement of teeth), or malocclusion.*

---

*The above-listed penalties and disqualifications apply to all British

BRITISH SHORTHAIR COLORS

White, black, blue, cream, black smoke, blue smoke, classic tabby pattern, mackerel tabby pattern, spotted tabby pattern, silver tabby, red tabby, brown tabby, blue tabby, cream tabby, tortoiseshell, calico dilute calico, blue-cream, and bi-color (black and white, blue and white, red and white, or cream and white).

British Shorthair allowable outcross breeds: None.

BURMESE

AUTHOR'S NOTE: The Burmese is a soft-spoken, active cat with a pleasing personality. These are playful cats with a lot of funny moves, from quick rollovers to prancing back and forth. They are gregarious and people-loving. Wong Mau of Burma was the mother of the entire American Burmese breed. She was brought to America in the 1930s and mated with a Siamese for lack of another Burmese. The Cat-Book Poems, *dating from the Ayudhya period of Siam (1350–1767), picture the Burmese on a page with the Siamese, the Korat, and a black cat with a white collar called the Singha-sep. All the descendants of this historic line of great cats have a sumptuous brown coat.*

CFA Show Standards

POINT SCORE

HEAD, EARS, AND EYES (30)

    Roundness of head 7
    Breadth between eyes and Full face 6
    Proper profile (includes Chin) 6
    Ear set, placement, and size 6
    Eye placement and shape 5

BODY, LEGS, FEET, AND TAIL (30)

    Torso 15
    Muscle tone 5

Shorthair cats. Additional penalties and disqualifications are listed under colors *[in "CFA Show Standards"].*

GENERAL: The overall impression of the ideal Burmese would be a cat of medium size with substantial bone structure, good muscular development, and a surprising weight for its size. This together with expressive eyes and a sweet expression presents a totally distinctive cat that is comparable to no other breed. Perfect physical condition, with excellent muscle tone. There should be no evidence of obesity, paunchiness, weakness, or apathy.

HEAD, EARS, and EYES: Head pleasingly rounded without flat planes whether viewed from the front or side. The face is full, with considerable breadth between the eyes, and blends gently into a broad, well-developed, short muzzle that maintains the rounded contours of the head. In profile there is a visible nose break. The chin is firmly rounded, reflecting a proper bite. The head sits on a well-developed neck. The ears are medium in size, set well apart, broad at the base, and rounded at the tips. Tilting slightly forward, the ears contribute to an alert appearance. The eyes are large, set far apart, with rounded aperture.

BODY: Medium in size, muscular in development, and presenting a compact appearance. Allowance to be made for larger size in males. An ample, rounded chest, with back level from shoulder to tail.

LEGS: Well proportioned to body.

PAWS: Round. Toes: five in front and four behind.

TAIL: Straight, medium in length.

COAT: Fine, glossy, satinlike texture; short and very close-lying.

PENALIZE: Distinct barring on either the front or rear outer legs. Trace (faint) barring permitted in kittens and young adults.

DISQUALIFY: Kinked or abnormal tail, lockets or spots. Blue eyes. Incorrect nose leather or paw pad color. Malocclusion of the jaw that results in a severe underbite or overbite that visually prohibits the described profile, and/or malformation that results in protruding teeth or a wry face or jaw. Distinct barring on the torso.

BURMESE COLORS

SABLE: The mature specimen is a rich, warm sable brown, shading almost imperceptibly to a slightly lighter hue on the underparts but otherwise without shadings, barring, or markings of any kind. (Kittens are often lighter in color.) **Nose leather and paw pads**—Brown. **Eye color**—Ranges from gold to yellow, the greater the depth and brilliance the better. Green eyes are a fault.

CHAMPAGNE: The mature specimen should be a warm honey-beige, shading to a pale gold tan underside. Slight darkening on ears and face permissible but lesser shading preferred. A slight darkening in older specimens allowed, the emphasis being on evenness of color. **Nose leather**—Light warm brown. **Paw pads**—Warm pinkish tan. **Eye color**—Ranging from yellow to gold, the greater the depth and brilliance the better.

BLUE: The mature specimen should be a medium blue with warm fawn undertones, shading almost imperceptibly to a slightly lighter hue on the underparts, but otherwise without shadings, barring, or markings of any kind. **Nose leather and paw pads**—Slate gray. **Eye color**—Ranging from yellow to gold, the greater the depth and brilliance the better.

PLATINUM: The mature specimen should be a pale, silvery gray with pale fawn undertones, shading almost imperceptibly to a slightly lighter hue on the underparts, but otherwise without shadings, barring, or markings of any kind. **Nose**

leather and paw pads—Lavender-pink. **Eye color**—Ranging from yellow to gold, the greater the depth and brilliance the better.

Burmese allowable outcross breeds: None.

CHARTREUX

AUTHOR'S NOTE: The Chartreux is a large, strapping cat that is gentle and good-natured (except when it comes to mice). These cats are friendly and quite amiable with all members of their family, including other pets and visitors. They are similar to the British Shorthair in size and appearance. These are among the oldest of cat breeds, having existed before they lived with the Carthusian monks of France in their mother house, "Le Grand Chartreux," in the seventeenth century.

CFA Show Standards

POINT SCORE

HEAD (35)
 Shape and size 6
 Profile/nose 5
 Muzzle 5
 Ear shape and size .5
 Ear placement 5
 Eye shape and size .5
 Neck 4
BODY (30)
 Shape and size 8
 Legs and feet 8
 Boning 5
 Musculature 5
 Tail 4
COAT (20)
 Texture 15
 Length 5
COLOR (19)
 Coat color 10
 Eye color 5

GENERAL: The Chartreux is a sturdy French breed coveted since antiquity for its hunting prowess and its dense, water-repellent fur. Its husky, robust type is sometimes termed primitive, neither cobby nor classic. Though amply built, Chartreux are extremely supple and agile cats; refined, never coarse or clumsy. Males are much larger than females and slower to mature. Coat texture, coat color, and eye color are affected by sex, age, and natural factors, which should not penalize. The qualities of strength, intelligence, and amenability, which have enabled the Chartreux to survive the centuries unaided, should be evident in all exhibition animals and preserved through careful selection.

HEAD and NECK: Rounded and broad but not a sphere. Powerful jaw; full cheeks, with mature males having larger jowls. High, softly contoured forehead; nose straight and of medium length/width, with a slight stop at eye level. Muzzle comparatively small, narrow, and tapered, with slight pads. Sweet, smiling expression. Neck short and heavy set.

EARS: Medium in height and width; set fairly high on the head; very erect posture.

EYES: Rounded and open; alert and expressive. Color range is copper to gold; a clear, deep, brilliant orange is preferred.

BODY and TAIL: Robust physique: medium-long with broad shoulders and deep chest. Strong boning; muscle mass is solid and dense. Females are medium; males are large. Tail of moderate length; heavy at base; tapering to oval tip. Lively and flexible.

LEGS and FEET: Legs of medium length; straight and sturdy; comparatively fine-boned. Feet are found and medium in size (may appear almost dainty compared to body mass).

COAT: Medium-short and slightly woolly in texture (should break like a sheepskin at neck and flanks). Resilient undercoat; longer, protective topcoat. NOTE: degree of woolliness depends on age, sex, and habitat, mature males exhibiting the heaviest coats. Silkier, thinner coat permitted on females and cats under two years.

PENALIZE: Severe nose break, snubbed or upturned nose, broad, heavy muzzle, palpable tail defect, eyes too close together, giving angry look.

DISQUALIFY: White locket, visible tail kink, green eyes.

CHARTREUX COLOR

COLOR: Any shade of blue-gray from ash to slate; tips lightly rushed with silver. Emphasis on color clarity and uniformity rather than shade. Preferred tone is a bright, unblemished blue with an overall iridescent sheen. Nose leather is slate gray; lips blue; paw pads are rose-taupe. Allowance made for ghost barring in kittens and for tail rings in juveniles under two years of age.

Chartreux allowable outcross breeds: None.

COLORPOINT SHORTHAIR

AUTHOR'S NOTE: Similar in personality to the Siamese, the Colorpoint Shorthair is an intelligent cat with an affectionate nature and a desire to please. Whether show cats or pets, these oriental beauties are almost like dogs in their physical desire to fetch, bow, and do other tricks, to talk to you as much as possible and to follow you around the house. The Colorpoint Shorthair appears to be a Siamese with colors other than the traditional Siamese point colors (i.e., Seal Point, Chocolate Point, Blue Point, and Lilac Point). CFA accepts the Colorpoint Shorthair as a separate breed, partly because traditional Siamese breeders do not wish to permit any colors other than the four traditional ones and partly because the breed was crossed with American Shorthairs to introduce the new colors. Complicating the issue further is the Oriental Shorthair, which is another nontraditional version of the Siamese. It does not have color points on the extremities of its body, but has a solid color over the entire body.

CFA Show Standards

POINT SCORE

HEAD (20)
    Long flat profile 6
    Wedge, fine muzzle, size 5
    Ears 4

GENERAL: A medium-size, refined, and svelte cat with long tapering lines; very lithe, but muscular. Males may be proportionately larger. Excellent physical condition, neither flabby nor bony. Eyes clear. Not fat.

HEAD: Long, tapering wedge. Medium in size, in good proportion to body. The total wedge starts at the nose and flares out in straight lines to the tips of the ears, forming an approximate equilateral triangle, with no break at the whiskers. No less than the width of an eye between the eyes. When the whiskers are smoothed back, the underlying bone structure is apparent. Allowance must be made for jowls in the stud cat.

SKULL: Flat. In profile, a long, straight line is seen from the top of the head to the tip of the nose. No bulge over eyes. No dip in nose.

NECK: Long and slender.

NOSE: Long and straight. A continuation of the forehead, with no break.

MUZZLE: Fine, wedge-shaped.

EARS: Strikingly large, pointed, wide at base, continuing the lines of the wedge.

EYES: Almond-shaped. Medium size. Neither protruding

nor recessed. Slanted toward the nose in harmony with lines of wedge and ears. Uncrossed. *[Eye color, deep vivid blue.]*

CHIN and JAW: Medium in size. Tip of chin lines with tip of nose in the same vertical plane. Neither receding nor excessively massive.

BODY: Medium size, long, and svelte. A distinctive combination of fine bones and firm muscles. Shoulders and hips continue same sleek lines of tubular body. Hips never wider than shoulders. Abdomen tight.

LEGS: Long and slim. Hind legs higher than front. In good proportion to body.

PAWS: Dainty, small, and oval. Toes: Five in front and four behind.

TAIL: Long, thin, tapering to a fine point.

COAT: Short, fine-textured, glossy. Lying close to body.

COLOR: **Body**—Subtle shading is permissible, but clear color is preferable. Allowance should be made for darker color in older cats, as Colorpoint Shorthairs generally darken with age, but there must be definite contrast between body color and points. **Points**—Mask, ears, feet, legs, and tail dense and clearly defined. All of the same shade. Mask covers entire face, including whisker pads, and is connected to ears by tracings. Mask should not extend over the top of the head. No white hairs in points.

PENALIZE: Pigmentation of nose leather and/or paw pads that is not consistent with the cat's particular color description. Palpable and/or visible protrusion of the cartilage at the end of the sternum.

DISQUALIFY: Any evidence of illness or poor health. Weak hind legs. Mouth breathing due to nasal obstruction or poor occlusion. Emaciation. Visible kink. Eyes other than blue. White toes and/or feet. Incorrect number of toes. Malocclusion resulting in either undershot or overshot chin.

COLORPOINT SHORTHAIR COLORS

Red point, cream point, seal lynx point, chocolate lynx point, blue lynx point, lilac lynx point, red lynx point, seal-tortie point, chocolate-tortie point, blue-cream point, lilac-cream point, seal-tortie lynx point, chocolate-tortie lynx point, blue-cream lynx point, lilac-cream lynx point, and cream lynx point.

Colorpoint Shorthair allowable outcross breeds: Siamese.

CORNISH REX

AUTHOR'S NOTE: Of course the most distinguishing feature of this unusual breed is its part wavy, part curly undercoat, which barely covers its delicate, tubular body. The coat has no guard hairs or topcoat, which exaggerates its ears and facial features. The breed has an extreme look that is just right for anyone desiring an unusual looking cat. In many ways the personality of the Cornish Rex and its close cousin, the Devon Rex, resembles the personality of the Siamese. It is intensely curious, affectionate, needful of human attention, and highly talkative. Once relaxed in their homes, these cats are extremely playful. One cannot mistake a Cornish Rex. They are small-to-medium, lean, curly-coated cats. They were the result of a spontaneous mutation born to Domestic Shorthairs during the 1950s. They appeared in England, Germany, and the United States. There are two recessive Rex genes, the Cornish and the Devon, that cannot breed together to produce a Rex. But both genes cause the cat to have a curly undercoat with no topcoat. Most cats have only a topcoat.

CFA Show Standards

POINT SCORE

HEAD (25)
Size and shape 5
Muzzle and Nose 5
Eyes 5
Ears 5
Profile 5
BODY (30)
Size 3
Torso 10

Legs and Paws 5
Tail 5
Bone 5
Neck 2
COAT (40)
Texture 10
Length 5
Wave, extent of wave 20
Close lying 5
COLOR 5

GENERAL: The Cornish Rex is distinguished from all other breeds by its extremely soft, wavy coat and racy type. It is surprisingly heavy and warm to the touch. All contours of the Cornish Rex are gently curved. By nature, the Cornish Rex is intelligent, alert, and generally likes to be handled.

PROFILE: A curve composed of two convex arcs. The forehead is rounded, the nose break smooth and mild, and the Roman nose has a high, prominent bridge.

HEAD: Comparatively small and narrow; length about one-third greater than the width. A definite whisker break. Gently curved outlines.

MUZZLE: Narrowing slightly to a rounded end.

EARS: Large and full from the base, erect and alert; set high on the head.

EYES: Medium to large in size, oval in shape, and slanting slightly upward. A full eye's width apart. Color should be clear, intense, and appropriate to coat color. *[Eye colors, deep blue, gold, brilliant gold, green, blue-green, or hazel.]*

NOSE: Roman. Length is one-third length of head. In profile a straight line from end of nose to chin, with considerable depth and squarish effect.

CHEEKS: Lean and muscular.

CHIN: Strong, well developed.

BODY: Small to medium, males proportionately larger. Torso long and slender, not tubular; hips, muscular and somewhat heavy in proportion to the rest of the body. Back is naturally arched, with lower line of the body approaching the upward curve. The arch is evident when the cat is standing naturally.

SHOULDERS: Well knit.

RUMP: Rounded, well muscled.

LEGS: Very long and slender. Hips well muscled, somewhat heavy in proportion to the rest of the body. The Cornish Rex stands high on its legs.

PAWS: Dainty, slightly oval. Toes, five in front and four behind.

TAIL: Long and slender, tapering toward the end and extremely flexible.

NECK: Long and slender.

BONE: Fine and delicate.

COAT: Short, extremely soft, silky, and completely free of guard hairs. Relatively dense. A tight, uniform marcel wave, lying close to the body and extending from the top of the head across the back, sides, and hips, continuing to the tip of the tail. Size and depth of wave may vary. The fur on the underside of the chin and on chest and abdomen is short and noticeably wavy.

CONDITION: Firm and muscular.

PENALIZE: Sparse coat or bare spots.

DISQUALIFY: Kinked or abnormal tail. Incorrect number of toes. Any coarse or guard hairs. Any signs of lameness in the hindquarters. Signs of poor health.

CORNISH REX COLORS

White, black, blue, red, cream, chinchilla silver, shaded silver, black smoke, blue smoke, classic tabby pattern, mackerel tabby pattern, patched tabby pattern, brown patched tabby, blue patched tabby, silver patched tabby, silver tabby (classic, mackerel), red tabby (classic, mackerel), brown tabby (classic, mackerel), blue tabby (classic, mackerel), cream tabby (classic, mackerel), tortoiseshell, calico, van calico, dilute calico, blue-cream, van blue-cream and white, bi-color (solid color and white, smoke and white, tabby and white, etc.), and van bi-color (black and white, red and white, blue and white, cream and white).

ORC (Other Rex Colors): Any other color or pattern. **Eye Color:** Appropriate to the predominant color of the cat.

Cornish Rex allowable outcross breeds: None.

CYMRIC

AUTHOR'S NOTE: To know the Manx is to know the Cymric. This breed is essentially a tailless Manx with long hair. Like Manx, Cymrics are often playful, good-natured, and affectionate with some, but not with others. These are bright, intelligent cats that are gentle and quiet. For many years the CFA registered the Cymric as a variety of Manx. It is only in recent years that the cat has been registered and shown as a separate breed. It is not considered a hybrid (man-made breed) because longhair kittens have often appeared in Manx litters for years. Both shorthair Manx parents must have the longhair gene to produce Cymric kittens. Cymric means ''of the Welsh.''

CFA Show Standards

POINT SCORE

Head and Ears 25
Eyes 5
Body 25
Taillessness 5
Legs and Feet 15
Coat Length 10
Coat Texture 10
Color 5

GENERAL: The overall impression of the tailless Cymric is that of roundness—round head with firm, round muzzle and prominent cheeks; broad chest; substantial short front legs; short back which arches from shoulders to a round rump; great depth of flank; and rounded, muscular thighs. The heavy, glossy double coat of medium length is the main differentiating factor of the Cymric from its parent breed, the Manx. The Cymric should be alert, clear of eye, with a glistening, clean, well-groomed coat. It should have a healthy physical appearance, feeling firm and muscular, neither too fat nor too lean. It should be surprisingly heavy when lifted. Cymrics are slow to mature, and allowance should be made in young cats.

HEAD and EARS: Round head with prominent cheeks and a jowly appearance. Head is slightly longer than it is broad. Moderately rounded forehead, pronounced cheekbones, and jowliness (more evident in adult males) enhance the round appearance. Short, thick neck. Definite whisker break, with large, round whisker pads. In profile there is a gentle nose dip. Well-developed muzzle, slightly longer than broad, with a strong chin. Ears are wide at the base, tapering gradually to a rounded tip, with full interior furnishings. Medium in size in proportion to the head, widely spaced, and set slightly outward. When viewed from behind, the ear set resembles that of the rocker of a cradle.

EYES: Large, round, and full. Set at a slight angle toward the nose (outer corners slightly higher than inner corners). Ideal color conforms to requirements of coat color. [*Eye colors, deep blue, brilliant copper, green, blue-green, or hazel.*]

BODY: Solidly muscled, compact and well balanced, medium in size, with sturdy bone structure. The Cymric is stout in appearance, with broad chest and well-sprung ribs; surprisingly heavy when lifted. The constant repetition of curves and circles gives the Cymric the appearance of great substance and durability, a cat that is powerful without the slightest hint of coarseness. Males may be somewhat larger than females.

Flank (fleshy area of the side, between the ribs and hip) has greater depth than in other breeds, causing considerable depth to the body when viewed from the side. The short back forms a smooth, continuous arch from shoulders to rump, curving at the rump to form the desirable round look. Shortness of back is unique to the Cymric (and Manx), but is in proportion to the entire cat and may be somewhat longer in the male. Because of the Cymric's longer coat over the rump area, the body may appear longer.

TAILLESSNESS: Absolute in the perfect specimen, with a decided hollow at the end of the backbone where, in the tailed cat, a tail would begin. A rise of the bone at the end of the spine is allowed and should not be penalized unless it is such that it stops the judge's hand, thereby spoiling the tailless appearance of the cat. The rump is extremely broad and round.

LEGS AND FEET: Heavily boned, forelegs short and set well apart to emphasize the broad, deep chest. Hind legs much longer than forelegs, with heavy, muscular thighs and substantial lower legs. Longer hind legs cause the rump to be considerably higher than the shoulders. Hind legs are straight when viewed from behind. Paws are neat and round, with five toes in front and four behind.

COAT LENGTH: The double coat is of medium length, dense and well padded over the main body, gradually lengthening from the shoulders to the rump. Breeches, abdomen, and neck ruff are longer than the main body. Cheek coat is thick and full. The collar-like neck ruff extends from the shoulders, being bib-like around the chest. Breeches should be full and thick to the hocks in the mature cat. Lower leg and head coat (except for cheeks) should be shorter than on the main body and neck ruff, but dense and full in appearance. Toe tufts and ear tufts are desirable. Preference should be given to the cat showing full coating.

COAT—TEXTURE: Coat is soft and silky, falling smoothly on the body yet being full and plush due to the double coat. Coat should have a healthy, glossy appearance. Allowance to be made for seasonal and age variations.

TRANSFER TO AOV: Definite, visible tail joint. Short coat.

PENALIZE: Coat that lacks density, has a cottony texture, or one that is of an overall even length.

SEVERELY PENALIZE: If the judge is unable to make the cat stand or walk properly.

DISQUALIFY: Evidence of poor physical condition, incorrect number of toes, evidence of hybridization.

CYMRIC COLORS

White, black, blue, red, cream, chinchilla silver, shaded silver, black smoke, blue smoke, classic tabby pattern, mackerel tabby pattern, patched tabby pattern, brown patched tabby, blue patched tabby, silver patched tabby, silver tabby (classic, mackerel), red tabby (classic, mackerel), brown tabby (classic, mackerel), blue tabby (classic, mackerel), cream tabby (classic, mackerel), tortoiseshell, calico, dilute calico, blue-cream, and bi-color (white with unbrindled patches of black, white with unbrindled patches of blue, white with unbrindled patches of red, or white with unbrindled patches of cream).

OCC (Other Cymric Colors): Any other color or pattern with the exception of those showing hybridization resulting in the colors chocolate, lavender, the Himalayan pattern, or these combinations with white. **Eye color**—Appropriate to the predominant color of the cat. *[Eye colors, deep blue, brilliant copper, green, blue-green, or hazel.]*

Cymric allowable outcross breeds: Manx.

DEVON REX

AUTHOR'S NOTE: The Devon Rex is understandably confused with the Cornish Rex because they are similar in appearance. However, they are two separate breeds according to the dictates of genetics. The Devon Rex was discovered ten years after the Cornish Rex, in Devon, England. Although both Rex breeds are similar in personality to the Siamese, there are differences. As a matter of fact, some believe there are slight personality differences between the two Rex breeds. The Devon may be less talkative than the other two. The Rex is a quiet lap cat with a personality as soft and cuddly as its fur. Both the Cornish and the Devon are easily recognized by their short, soft, tightly curled coat; long, slim, and agile body; narrow head; oval-shaped eyes, which slant upward; and long Roman nose.

CFA Show Standards

POINT SCORE

HEAD (35)

    Size and Shape 10

    Muzzle and Chin 5

    Profile 5

    Eyes 5

    Ears 10

BODY (30)

    Torso 10

    Legs and Paws 10

    Tail 5

    Neck 5

COAT (30)

    Density 10

    Texture and length 10

    Waviness 10

COLOR 5

GENERAL: The Devon Rex is a breed of unique appearance. Its large eyes, short muzzle, prominent cheekbones, and huge, low-set ears create a characteristic elfin look. A cat of medium-fine frame, the Devon is well covered with soft, wavy fur; the fur is of a distinctive texture, as the mutation that causes the wavy coat is cultivated in no other breed. The Devon is alert and active and shows a lively interest in its surroundings.

HEAD: Modified wedge. In the front view, the wedge is delineated by a narrowing series of three (3) distinct convex curves: outer edge of ears, cheekbones, and whisker pads. Face to be full-cheeked, with pronounced cheekbones and a whisker break. In profile, nose with a strongly marked stop; forehead curving back to a flat skull.

MUZZLE: Short, well-developed. Prominent whisker pads.

CHIN: Strong, well-developed.

EYES: Large and wide set, oval in shape, and sloping toward outer edges of ears. Color should be clear, intense, and appropriate to coat color.

EARS: Strikingly large and set very low, very wide at the base, so that the outside base of ear extends beyond the line of the wedge. Tapering to rounded tops and well covered with fine fur. With or without earmuffs and/or ear-tip tufts.

BODY: Hard and muscular, slender, and of medium length. Broad in chest and medium-fine in boning, with medium-fine but sturdy legs. Carried high on the legs, with the hind legs somewhat longer than the front. Allowance to be made for larger size in males, as long as good proportions are maintained.

LEGS and PAWS: Legs long and slim. Paws small and oval, with five toes in front and four behind.

TAIL: Long, fine, and tapering, well covered with short fur.

NECK: Medium long and slender.

COAT: **Density**—The cat is well covered with fur, with the greatest density occurring on the back, sides, tail, legs, face, and ears. Slightly less density is permitted on the top of head, neck, chest, and abdomen. Bare patches are a fault in kittens and a serious fault in adults; however the existence of down on the underparts of the body should not be misinterpreted as bareness. Sparse hair on the temples (forehead in front of the ears) is not a fault. **Texture**—The coat is soft, fine, full-bodied, and Rexed (i.e., appearing to be without guard hairs). **Length**—The coat is short on the back, sides, upper legs, and tail. It is very short on the head, ears, neck, paws, chest, and abdomen. **Waviness**—A rippled wave effect should be apparent when the coat is smoothed with one's hand. The wave is most evident where the coat is the longest, on the body and tail.

PENALIZE: Narrow, long, or domestic-type shorthair head; small or high-set ears; short, bare, or bushy tail; straight or shaggy coat; bare patches.

DISQUALIFY: Extensive baldness, kinked or abnormal tail, incorrect number of toes, crossed eyes, weak hind legs. Any evidence of illness or poor health.

DEVON REX COLORS

White, black, blue, red, cream, chocolate, lavender, cinnamon, fawn, shaded silver, blue shaded, chocolate shaded, lavender shaded, cameo shaded, cinnamon shaded, fawn shaded, tortoiseshell shaded, blue-cream shaded, chocolate tortoiseshell shaded, cinnamon tortoiseshell shaded, lavender-cream shaded, fawn-cream shaded, chinchilla, black smoke, blue smoke, red smoke cameo (cameo), chocolate smoke, lavender smoke, cinnamon smoke, cream smoke, fawn smoke, tortoiseshell smoke, blue-cream smoke, chocolate tortoiseshell smoke, lavender-cream smoke, cinnamon tortoiseshell smoke, fawn-cream smoke, classic tabby pattern, mackerel tabby pattern, spotted tabby pattern, patched tabby pattern, silver tabby, brown tabby, blue tabby, red tabby, cream tabby, chocolate (chestnut) tabby, chocolate silver tabby, cinnamon tabby, cinnamon silver tabby, lavender tabby, lavender silver tabby, fawn tabby, cameo tabby, blue silver-, cream silver-, and fawn silver-tabbies, tortoiseshell, blue-cream, chocolate (chestnut) tortoiseshell, cinnamon tortoiseshell, lavender-cream, fawn-cream, calico (white with unbrindled patches of black and red), van calico (white cat with unbrindled patches of black and red confined to the extremities), dilute calico, dilute van calico, bi-color (solid color and white, tabby and white, tortoiseshell and white, etc.), van bi-color (solid color and white, tabby and white, tortoiseshell and white, etc.), fawn-cream calico, lavender-cream calico, and cinnamon-cream calico.

ODRC (Other Devon Rex Colors): Any other color or pattern. Cats with no more than a locket and/or button do not qualify for this class; such cats shall be judged in the color class of their basic color with no penalty for such locket and/or button. Examples—Any color with one, two, three, or four white feet. Ticked tabbies. All point-restricted colors such as seal point, chocolate point, blue point, lilac point, cream point, lynx points, cinnamon point, etc.

Devon Rex allowable outcross breeds: American Shorthair or British Shorthair for litters born before 5/1/98.

EGYPTIAN MAU

AUTHOR'S NOTE: Although this breed has been accepted for registration and showing since the late 1970s, it is still quite rare. The Egyptian Mau personality varies from cat to cat, between aloofness and sociability. Generally, they are affectionate with their own families but reserved with strangers. The Mau retains a hint of the wild from which it most likely came. It has that supposedly typical cat quality of aloof reserve, making close friends with only a special few. Physically, it strikes a delicate balance between the compactness of a Burmese and the slim elegance of a Siamese. The coat pattern and color of the Mau are its most distinctive features, with random spots dotted over a silver, bronze, or smoke ground color. Its "gooseberry green" eyes stare out like liquid neon. Like its cousin, the more active Abyssinian, it has a birdlike vocal quality that is both soft and mellow. It is a rare cat, indeed.

CFA Show Standards

POINT SCORE

HEAD (20)
  Muzzle 5
  Skull 5
  Ears 5
  Eye shape 5
BODY (25)
  Torso 10
  Legs and Feet 10
  Tail 5
COAT (5)
  Texture and length 5
PATTERN (25)
COLOR (25)
  Eye color 10
  Coat color 15

GENERAL: The Egyptian Mau is the only natural domesticated breed of spotted cat. The Egyptian's impression should be one of an active, colorful cat of medium size with well-developed muscles. Perfect physical condition with an alert appearance. Well balanced physically and temperamentally. Males tend to be larger than females.

HEAD: A slightly rounded wedge without flat planes, medium in length. Not full-cheeked. Profile showing a gentle contour, with slight rise from the bridge of the nose to the forehead. Entire length of nose even in width when viewed from the front.

MUZZLE: Neither short nor pointed. Allowance to be made for jowls in adult males.

EARS: Medium to large, alert and moderately pointed, continuing the planes of the head. Broad at base. Upstanding, with ample width between ears. Hair in ears short and close-lying. Inner ear a delicate, almost transparent, shell pink. May be tufted.

EYES: Large and alert, almond-shaped, with a slight slant toward the ears. Skull apertures neither round nor oriental.

BODY: Medium long and graceful, showing well-developed muscular strength. Loose skin flap extending from flank to hind-leg knee. General balance is more to be desired than size alone. Allowance to be made for muscular necks and shoulders in adult males.

LEGS and FEET: In proportion to body. Hind legs proportionately longer, giving the appearance of being on tiptoe when standing upright. Feet small and dainty, slightly oval, almost round in shape. Toes, five in front and four behind.

TAIL: Medium long, thick at base, with slight taper.

COAT: Hair is medium in length with a lustrous sheen. In the smoke color, the hair is silky and fine in texture. In the silver and bronze colors, the hair is dense and resilient in texture and accommodates two or more bands of ticking, separated by lighter bands.

PENALIZE: Short or round head. Pointed muzzle. Small, round, or oriental eyes. Cobby or oriental body. Short or whip tail. If no broken necklaces. Pencilings in spotting pattern on torso. Poor condition. Amber cast in eye color in cats over the age of one year.

DISQUALIFY: Lack of spots. Blue eyes. Kinked or abnormal tail. Incorrect number of toes. White locket or button distinctive from other acceptable white-colored areas in color sections of standard.

MAU PATTERN
(COMMON TO ALL COLORS)

PATTERN: Markings on torso are to be randomly spotted, with variance in size and shape. The spots can be small or large, round, oblong, or irregularly shaped. Any of these are of equal merit, but the spots, however shaped or whatever size, shall be distinct. Good contrast between pale ground color and deeper markings. Forehead barred with characteristic "M" and frown marks, forming lines between the ears which continue down the back of the neck, ideally breaking into elongated spots, along the spine. As the spinal lines reach the rear haunches, they meld together to form a dorsal stripe which continues along the top of the tail to its tip. The tail is heavily banded and has a dark tip. The cheeks are barred with "mascara" lines; the first starts at the outer corner of the eye and continues along the contour of the cheek, with a second line, which starts at the center of the cheek and curves upward, almost meeting it below the base of the ear. On the upper chest there are one or more broken necklaces. The shoulder markings are a transition between stripes and spots. The upper front legs are heavily barred but do not necessarily match. Spotting pattern on each side of the torso need not match. Haunches and upper hind legs to be a transition between stripes and spots, breaking into bars on the lower leg. Underside of body to have "vest buttons" spots; dark in color against the correspondingly pale ground color.

EGYPTIAN MAU COLORS

EYE COLOR: Light green ("gooseberry green"). Amber cast is acceptable only in young adults up to 1½ years of age.

BRONZE: Warm coppery brown ground color across head,

shoulders, outer legs, back, and tail, being darkest on the saddle and lightening to a tawny buff on the sides. Underside fades to a creamy ivory. All markings dark brown-black with a warm coppery brown undercoat, showing good contrast against the lighter ground color. Back of ears tawny pink and tipped in dark brown-black. Nose, lips, and eyes outlined in dark brown, with bridge of nose brown. Upper throat area, chin, and around nostrils pale creamy white. **Nose leather**—Brick red. **Paw pads**—Black or dark brown, with same color between toes and extending beyond the paws of the hind legs.

SILVER: Pale silver ground color across the head, shoulders, outer legs, back, and tail. Underside fades to a brilliant pale silver. All markings charcoal color with a white to pale silver undercoat, showing good contrast against lighter ground colors. Back of ears grayish-pink and tipped in black. Nose, lips, and eyes outlined in black. Upper throat area, chin, and around nostrils pale clear silver, appearing white. **Nose leather**—Brick red. **Paw pads**—Black with black between the toes and extending beyond the paws of the hind legs.

SMOKE: Pale silver ground color across head, shoulders, legs, tail, and underside. All markings jet black with a white-to-pale-silver undercoat, with sufficient contrast against ground color for pattern to be plainly visible. Nose, lips, and eyes outlined in jet black. Upper throat area, chin, and around nostrils lightest in color. **Nose leather**—Black. **Paw pads**—Black with black between the toes and extending beyond the paws of the hind legs.

Egyptian Mau allowable outcross breeds: None.

EXOTIC SHORTHAIR

AUTHOR'S NOTE: The Exotic Shorthair looks like a Persian with short hair. In the 1960s the Persian was crossed with the American Shorthair. The result was a sweet, gentle cat with a sharp wit and a plush coat. For all intents and purposes, this cat is a Persian that is easy to groom. Exotics have a sweet disposition and a talent for finding the best places to lounge around and sleep. For many, they are the ideal pet, with their massive Persian look and low-maintenance coats.

CFA Show Standards

POINT SCORE

Head (including size and shape of eyes; ear shape and
set) 30
Type (including shape, size, bone, and length of tail) . . 20
Coat 10
Balance 5
Refinement 5
Color 20
Eye Color 10

In all tabby varieties, the 20 points for color are to be divided 10 for markings and 10 for color. In all "with white" varieties (calico, dilute calico, bi-color, van bi-color, van calico, van dilute calico, and tabby and white), the 20 points for color are to be divided 10 for "with white" pattern and 10 for color.

GENERAL: The ideal Exotic Shorthair should present an impression of a heavily boned, well-balanced cat with a sweet expression and soft, round lines. The large, round eyes set wide apart in a large, round head contribute to the overall look and expression. The thick, plush coat softens the lines of the cat and accentuates the roundness in appearance.

HEAD: Round and massive, with great breadth of skull. Round face with round underlying bone structure. Well set on a short, thick neck.

NOSE: Short, snub, and broad. With "break."

CHEEKS: Full.

JAWS: Broad and powerful.

CHIN: Full, well developed, and firmly rounded, reflecting a proper bite.

EARS: Small, round-tipped, tilted forward, and not unduly open at the base. Set far apart, and low on the head, fitting into (without distorting) the rounded contour of the head.

EYES: Brilliant in color, large, round, and full. Set level and far apart, giving a sweet expression to the face.

BODY: Of cobby type, low on the legs, broad and deep through the chest, equally massive across the shoulders and rump, with a well-rounded mid-section and level back. Good muscle tone, with no evidence of obesity. Large or medium in size. Quality the determining consideration rather than size.

LEGS: Short, thick, and strong. Forelegs straight.

PAWS: Large, round, and firm. Toes carried close, five in front and four behind.

TAIL: Short, but in proportion to body length. Carried without a curve and at an angle lower than the back.

COAT: Dense, plush, soft, and full of life. Standing out from the body due to dense undercoat. Medium in length. Acceptable length depends on proper undercoat. Penalize for a flat or close-lying coat that falls over due to lack of support by a rich, thick undercoat. Cats with a ruff or tail-feathers (long hair on the tail) shall be transferred to the AOV class.

DISQUALIFY: Locket or button. Kinked or abnormal tail. Incorrect number of toes. Any apparent weakness in the hindquarters. Any apparent deformity of the spine. Deformity of the skull resulting in an asymmetrical face and/or head. Crossed eyes. For pointed cats, disqualify for white toes, eye color other than blue.*

EXOTIC SHORTHAIR COLORS

White, black, blue, red, cream, chocolate, lilac, chinchilla silver, shaded silver, chinchilla golden, shaded golden, shell cameo (red chinchilla), shaded cameo (red shaded), shell tortoiseshell, shaded tortoiseshell, black smoke, blue smoke, cameo smoke (red smoke), smoke tortoiseshell, blue-cream smoke, classic tabby pattern, mackerel tabby pattern, patched tabby, brown patched tabby, blue patched tabby, silver patched tabby, silver tabby (classic, mackerel), red tabby (classic,

*The above-listed disqualifications apply to all Exotic Shorthair cats. Additional disqualifications are listed under "Colors," in CFA "Show Standards."

mackerel), brown tabby (classic, mackerel), blue tabby (classic, mackerel), cream tabby (classic, mackerel), cameo tabby (classic, mackerel), peke-face red and peke-face red tabby, tortoiseshell, calico, dilute calico, blue-cream, bi-color (black and white, blue and white, red and white, or cream and white), van bi-color, van calico, van dilute calico, tabby and white, seal point, chocolate point, blue point, lilac point, lilac-cream point flame (red) point, cream point, tortie point, chocolate-tortie point, blue-cream, seal lynx point, blue lynx point, tortie-lynx point, and blue-cream lynx point.

Exotic Shorthair allowable outcross breeds: Persian.

HAVANA BROWN

AUTHOR'S NOTE: Sweet and loving cats, the Havana Brown draws its personality from the best breeds to combine a rich blend of intelligence and devotion. These cats are affectionate and playful and make ideal pets. The Havana Brown is actually brown. It was arduously bred in the 1950s from Siamese, Russian Blues, and black Domestic Shorthairs to achieve that beautiful brown coat and foreign body type (Siamese look). This is a bright, active cat that looks much like a Burmese. Its coat is a deep mahogany-toned brown resembling cured tobacco, deep down to its roots. Even its whiskers are brown.

CFA Show Standards

POINT SCORE

HEAD (33)
    Shape 8
    Profile/Stop 8
    Muzzle 8
    Chin 4
    Ears 5
EYES (10)
    Shape and Size 5
    Color 5
COLOR (22)

GENERAL: The overall impression of the ideal Havana Brown is a cat of medium size with a rich, solid-color coat and good muscle tone. Due to its distinctive muzzle shape, coat color, brilliant and expressive eyes, and large, forward-tilted ears, it is comparable to no other breed.

HEAD: When viewed from above, the head is longer than it is wide, narrowing to a rounded muzzle with a pronounced break on both sides, behind the whisker pads. The somewhat narrow muzzle and the whisker break are distinctive characteristics of the breed and must be evident in the typical specimen. When viewed in profile, there is a distinct stop at the eyes; the end of the muzzle appears almost square; this illusion is heightened by a well-developed chin, the profile outline of which is more square than round. Ideally, the tip of the nose and the chin form an almost perpendicular line. Allowance to be made for somewhat broader heads and stud jowls in the adult male. Allow for sparse hair on chin, directly below lower lip.

EARS: Large, round-tipped, cupped at the base, wide-set but not flaring; tilted forward, giving the cat an alert appearance. Little hair inside or outside.

EYES: Shape, aperture oval in shape. Medium size; set wide apart; brilliant, alert, and expressive. Color, any vivid and level shade of green; the deeper the color the better.

BODY and NECK: Torso medium in length, firm and muscular. Adult males tend to be larger than their female counterparts. Overall balance and proportion rather than size to be determining factor. The neck is medium in length and in proportion to the body. The general conformation is mid-range between the short-coupled, thick-set, and svelte breeds.

LEGS and FEET: The ideal specimen stands relatively high on its legs for a cat of medium proportions in trunk and tail. Legs are straight. The legs of females are slim and dainty; slenderness and length of leg will be less evident in the more powerfully muscled, mature males. Hind legs slightly longer than front. Paws are oval and compact. Toes, five in front and four behind.

TAIL: Medium in length and in proportion to the body; slender, neither whiplike nor blunt; tapering at the end. Not too broad at the base.

COAT: Short to medium in length, smooth and lustrous.

DISQUALIFY: Kinked tail, locket or button, incorrect number of toes, any eye color other than green, incorrect color of whiskers, nose leather or paw pads.

HAVANA BROWN COLOR

COLOR: A rich and even shade of warm brown throughout; color tends toward red-brown (mahogany) rather than black-brown. **Nose leather**—Brown with a rosy flush. **Paw pads**—Rosy toned. **Whiskers**—Brown, complementing the coat color. ALLOW FOR GHOST TABBY MARKINGS IN KITTENS AND YOUNG ADULTS.

Havana Brown allowable outcross breeds: None.

JAPANESE BOBTAIL

AUTHOR'S NOTE: The Japanese Bobtail personality is somewhat serious, with random episodes of playfulness. It is an active cat that always seems to be busy with something important to do. It is a devoted family pet that loves you but from a bit of a distance. These are congenial animals with a keen intelligence. Japan has had a cat for centuries on the streets, in the houses and temples, and recorded in the art of Japanese culture. It is a Japanese Bobtail. The Japanese love the tricolors best because they bring good luck. They call them Mi-Ki and keep little good-luck replicas of them with a paw raised. These cats can be recognized by their charming personalities, their somewhat slanted eyes, and, of course, by their bobbed tails, which can be any shape imaginable.

CFA Show Standards

POINT SCORE

HEAD 20
TYPE 30
TAIL 20
COLOR and MARKINGS 20
COAT 10

GENERAL: The Japanese Bobtail should present the overall impression of a medium-size cat with clean lines and bone structure, well muscled but straight and slender, rather than massive, in build. The unique set of its eyes, combined with high cheekbones and a long, parallel nose, lend a distinctive Japanese cast to the face, especially in profile, quite different from the other oriental breeds. Its short tail should resemble a bunny tail, with the hair fanning out to create a pom-pom appearance, which effectively camouflages the underlying bone structure of the tail.

HEAD: Although the head appears long and finely chiseled, it forms almost a perfect equilateral triangle (the triangle does not include the ears), with gentle curving lines, high cheekbones, and a noticeable whisker break, the nose long and well defined by two parallel lines from tip to brow with a gentle dip at, or just below, eye level. Allowance must be made for jowls in the stud cat.

EARS: Large, upright, and expressive, set wide apart but at right angles to the head rather than flaring outward, and giving the impression of being tilted forward in repose.

MUZZLE: Fairly broad and rounding into the whisker break; neither point nor blunt.

EYES: Large, oval rather than round, but wide and alert; set into the skull at a rather pronounced slant when viewed in profile. The eyeball shows a shallow curvature and should not bulge out beyond the cheekbone or the forehead.

BODY: Medium in size; males proportionately larger than

females. Torso long, lean, and elegant, not tubular, showing well-developed muscular strength without coarseness. No inclination toward flabbiness or cobbiness. General balance of utmost importance.

LEGS: In keeping with the body, long, slender, and high, but not dainty or fragile in appearance. The hind legs noticeably longer than the forelegs, but deeply angulated to bend when the cat is standing relaxed, so that the torso remains nearly level rather than rising toward the rear. When standing, the cat's forelegs and shoulders form two continuous straight lines, close together.

PAWS: Oval. Toes, five in front and four behind.

COAT: Medium length, soft and silky, but without a noticeable undercoat.

TAIL: The tail is unique not only to the breed, but to each individual cat. This is to be used as a guideline, rather than promoting one specific type of tail out of the many that occur within the breed.

The tail must be clearly visible and is composed of one or more curves, angles, or kinks or any combination thereof. The farthest extension of the tailbone from the body should be no longer than three inches. The direction in which the tail is carried is not important. The tail may be flexible or rigid and should be of a size and shape that harmonizes with the rest of the cat.

COLOR: In the bi-colors and tri-colors (Mi-Ke), any color may predominate, with preference given to bold, dramatic markings and vividly contrasting colors. In the solid-color cat, the coat color should be of uniform density and color from the tip to the root of each hair and from the nose of the cat to the tail. Nose leather, paw pads, and eye color should harmonize generally with coat color. Blue eyes and odd eyes are allowed.

PENALIZE: Short, round head, cobby build.

DISQUALIFY: Tailbone absent or extending too far beyond body. Tail lacking in pom-pom or fluffy appearance. Delayed bobtail effect (i.e., the pom-pom being preceded by an inch or two of normal tail with close-lying hair rather than appearing to commence at the base of the spine).

White, black, red, black and white, red and white, mi-ke (tri-color—black, red, and white), tortoiseshell (black, red, and cream).

OJBC (OTHER JAPANESE BOBTAIL COLORS): Include the following categories and any other color or pattern or combination thereof except coloring that is point-restricted (e.g., Siamese markings) or unpatterned agouti (e.g., Abyssinian coloring). "Patterned" categories denote and include any variety of tabby striping or spotting, with or without areas of solid (unmarked) color, with preference given to bold, dramatic markings and rich, vivid coloring.

Other solid colors—Blue or cream. Patterned self-colors—Red, black, blue, cream, silver, or brown. Other bi-colors—Blue and white or cream and white. Patterned bi-colors—Red, black, blue, cream, silver, or brown combined with white. Patterned tortoiseshell—Blue-cream. Patterned blue-cream. Dilute tri-colors: Blue, cream, and white. Patterned dilute tri-colors: Patterned mi-ke (tri-color), tortoiseshell with white.

Japanese Bobtail allowable outcross breeds: None.

JAVANESE

AUTHOR'S NOTE: The Javanese is essentially the same breed as the Balinese, which is to say it is a long-haired Siamese. However, CFA registers it as a separate breed. The difference between the Javanese and the Balinese is in the wide variety of coat colors allowed the Javanese by CFA (excluding the four traditional Siamese point colors). Javanese personalities are similar to those of all Siamese cats. They are very vocal and demanding of human attention. These are good-natured cats with an unquenchable curiosity. They insist on participating in all human activities. See Balinese and Siamese for more information.

CFA Show Standards

POINT SCORE

HEAD (20)
Long flat profile 6
Wedge, fine muzzle, size 5
Ears 4
Chin 3
Width between eyes 2

EYES (5)
Shape, size, slant, and placement 5

BODY (30)
Structure and size, including neck 12
Muscle tone 10
Legs and Feet 5
Tail 3

COAT (20)
Length 10
Texture 10

COLOR (25)
Body color 10
Point color (matching points of dense color, proper
foot pads and nose leather.) 10
Eye color 5

GENERAL: The ideal Javanese is a svelte cat with long, tapering lines, very lithe but strong and muscular. Excellent physical condition. Neither flabby nor bony. Not fat. Eyes clear. Because of the longer fur, the Javanese appears to have softer lines and less extreme type than other breeds of cats with similar type.

HEAD: Long, tapering wedge. Medium size, in good proportion to body. The total wedge starts at the nose and flares out in straight lines to the tips of the ears, forming a triangle, with no break at the whiskers. No less than the width of an eye between the eyes. When the whiskers and face hair are smoothed back, the underlying bone structure is apparent. Allowance must be made for jowls in the stud cat.

SKULL: Flat. In profile, a long, straight line is seen from the top of the head to the tip of the nose. No bulge over the eyes. No dip in nose.

NOSE: Long and straight. A continuation of the forehead with no break.

MUZZLE: Fine, wedge-shaped.

CHIN and JAW: Medium size. Tip of chin lines up with tip of nose in the same vertical plane. Neither receding nor excessively massive.

EARS: Strikingly large, pointed, wide at base, continuing the lines of the wedge.

EYES: Almond-shaped. Medium size. Neither protruding nor recessed. Slanted toward the nose in harmony with lines of wedge and ears. Uncrossed.

BODY: Medium size. Dainty, long, and svelte. A distinctive combination of fine bones and firm muscles. Shoulders and hips continue same sleek lines of tubular body. Hips never wider than shoulders. Abdomen tight. The male may be somewhat larger than the female.

NECK: Long and slender.

LEGS: Long and slim. Hind legs higher than front. In good proportion to body.

PAWS: Dainty, small, and oval. Toes: five in front and four behind.

TAIL: Bone structure long, thin, tapering to a fine point. Tail hair spreads out like a plume.

COAT: Long, fine, silky, without downy undercoat.

COLOR: **Body**—Even, with subtle shading when allowed. Allowance should be made for darker color in older cats, as Javanese generally darken with age, but there must be definite contrast between body color points. **Points**—Mask, ears, legs, feet, tail dense and clearly defined. All of the same shade. Mask covers entire face, including whisker pads, and is connected to ears by tracings. Mask should not extend over top of head. No ticking or white hairs in points.

PENALIZE: Lack of pigment in the nose leather and/or paw pads in part or in total. Crossed eyes.

DISQUALIFY: Any evidence of illness or poor health. Weak hind legs. Mouth breathing due to nasal obstruction or poor occlusion. Emaciation. Kink in tail. Eyes other than blue. White toes and/or feet. Incorrect number of toes. Definite double coat (i.e., downy undercoat).

JAVANESE COLORS

Red point, cream point, seal lynx point, chocolate lynx point, blue lynx point, lilac lynx point, red lynx point, chocolate-tortie lynx point, blue-cream lynx point, lilac-cream lynx point, cream lynx point, seal-tortie lynx point, seal-tortie point, chocolate-tortie point, blue-cream point, and lilac-cream point.

Javanese allowable outcross breeds: Balinese, Colorpoint Shorthair, or Siamese for litters born after May 1, 1995.

KORAT

AUTHOR'S NOTE: The Korat is a quiet cat with soft vocalizations. It will respond playfully to human attention and is very friendly. Family life is much to its liking, and strong relationships develop quickly. This intelligent feline enjoys its many naps throughout the day. These silver-blue cats are the native cat of the Korat province of Thailand. They are often called by their native Thai name, Si-Sawat, *which means "a cat with the color of the* Look-Sawat," *a wild fruit plant whose seed is a silver-blue color. Like the Japanese Bobtails, they are considered good luck. Sometime before the eighteenth century the Korat was described and pictured in* The Cat-Book Poems, *now in the Bangkok National Museum. It is one of the oldest recorded breeds in history. The breed was recognized by CFA for registration and showing in 1967. It is seen only in solid silver-blue, tipped with silver. The silver tipping creates a halo effect when the light is right.*

CFA Show Standards

POINT SCORE

HEAD (25)

Broad head 5
Profile 4
Breadth between eyes 4
Ear set and placement 4
Heartshape 5
Chin and Jaw 3

EYES (15)

Size 5
Shape 5
Placement 5

BODY (25)

Body 15
Legs and Feet 5
Tail 5

COAT (10)

Short 4
Texture 3
Close-lying 3

COLOR (25)

Body Color 20
Eye Color 5

GENERAL: The Korat is a rare cat even in Thailand, its country of origin, and because of its unusually fine disposition, it is greatly loved by the Thai people, who regard it as a 'good luck' cat. Its general appearance is of a silver-blue cat with a heavy silver sheen, medium-size, hard-bodied, and muscular. All smooth curves with huge eyes, luminous, alert, and expressive. Perfect physical condition, alert appearance.

HEAD: When viewed from the front, or looking down from just back of the head, the head is heartshaped, with breadth between and across the eyes. The eyebrow ridges form the upper curves of the heart, and the sides of the face gently curve down to the chin to complete the heartshape. Undesirable—any pinch or narrowness, especially between or across the eyes.

PROFILE: Well-defined with a slight stop between forehead and nose, which has a lion-like downward curve just above the leather. Undesirable—nose that appears either long or short in proportion.

CHIN and JAW: Strong and well-developed, making a balancing line for the profile and properly completing the heartshape. Neither overly squared nor sharply pointed, nor a weak chin that gives the head a pointed look.

EARS: Large, with a rounded tip and large flare at base, set high on head, giving an alert expression. Inside ears sparsely furnished. Hairs on outside of ears extremely short and close.

BODY: Semi-cobby, neither compact nor svelte. The torso is distinctive. Broad-chested with good space between forelegs. Muscular, supple, with a feeling of hard coiled-spring power and unexpected weight. Back is carried in a curve. The males tend to be larger than the females.

LEGS: Well-proportioned to body. Distance along back from nape of neck to base of tail appears to be equal to distance from base of tail to floor. Front legs slightly shorter than back legs.

PAWS: Oval. Toes: five in front and four behind.

TAIL: Medium in length, heavier at the base, tapering to a rounded tip. Non-visible kink permitted.

EYES: Large and luminous. Particularly prominent, with an extraordinary depth and brilliance. Wide open and oversize for the face. Eye aperture, which shows as well-rounded when fully open, has an Asian slant when closed or partially closed. Undesirable—small or dull-looking eyes.

COAT: Single. Hair is short in length, glossy and fine, lying close to the body. The coat over the spine is inclined to break as the cat moves.

DISQUALIFY: Visible kink. Incorrect number of toes. White spot or locket. Any color but silver blue.

KORAT COLOR

COLOR: Silver blue all over, tipped with silver; the silver should be sufficient to produce a silver halo effect. The hair is usually lighter at the roots, with a gradient of blue that is deepest just before the tips, which are silver. Without shading or tabby markings. Where the coat is short, the sheen of the silver is intensified. Undesirable: Coats with silver tipping on only the head, legs, and feet. **Nose leather and lips**—Dark blue or lavender. **Paw pads**—Dark blue ranging to lavender with a pinkish tinge. **Eye color**—Luminous green preferred; amber cast acceptable. Kittens and adolescents have yellow to amber-to-amber-green eyes. Color is not usually true until the cat is mature, usually two to four years of age.

Korat allowable outcross breeds: None.

MAINE COON CAT

AUTHOR'S NOTE: This true American breed is an impressive cat in every way. In addition to its large, handsome body, it has a pleasing personality of self-confidence, assertiveness, and calm playfulness. The Maine Coon Cat adjusts to other cats and even dogs with ease and comfort but tends to dominate most situations. Despite its slight voice, it is a formidable hunter. No cat ever mated with a raccoon, but the Maine Coon Cat often looks as if it did. The brown tabby varieties have rings on their big bushy tails, like raccoons'. The Maine Coon Cat, a natural breed, has come to be accepted as an indigenous American cat. Prized by New Englanders as being the largest, smartest, and most beautiful cat anywhere, the amiable Maine Coon is thought to be the by-product of shorthaired domestic cats, brought to the United States by the Pilgrims in 1640, and Angora cats, brought by seafaring New Englanders to these shores in the 1800s.

CFA Show Standards

POINT SCORE

HEAD (30)
  Shape 15
  Ears 10
  Eyes 5
BODY (35)
  Shape 20
  Neck 5
  Legs and Feet 5
  Tail 5
COAT 20
COLOR (15)
  Body color 10
  Eye color 5

GENERAL: Originally a working cat, the Maine Coon is solid, rugged, and can endure a harsh climate. A distinctive characteristic is its smooth, shaggy coat. With an essentially amiable disposition, it has adapted to varied environments.

HEAD SHAPE: Medium in width and medium-long in length, with a squareness to the muzzle. Allowance should be made for broadening in older studs. Cheekbones high. Chin firm and in line with nose and upper lip. Nose medium-long in length; slight concavity when viewed in profile.

EARS: Large, well-tufted, wide at base, tapering to appear pointed. Set high and well apart.

EYES: Large, expressive, wide-set. Slightly oblique setting, with slant toward outer base of ear.

NECK: Medium-long.

BODY SHAPE: Muscular, broad-chested. Size medium to large. Females generally are smaller than males. The body should be long, with all parts in proportion, to create a well-balanced rectangular appearance, with no part of the anatomy being so exaggerated as to foster weakness. Allowance should be made for slow maturation.

LEGS and FEET: Legs substantial, wide-set, of medium length, and in proportion to the body. Paws large, round, well-tufted. Five toes in front; four in back.

TAIL: Long, wide at base, and tapering. Fur long and flowing.

COAT: Heavy and shaggy; shorter on the shoulders and longer on the stomach and britches. Frontal ruff desirable. Texture silky, with coat falling smoothly.

PENALIZE: A coat that is short or overall even.

DISQUALIFY: Delicate bone structure. Undershot chin. Crossed eyes. Kinked tail. Incorrect number of toes. Buttons, lockets, or spots.

MAINE COON CAT COLORS

COAT COLOR: White, black, blue, red, and cream, silver tabby, red tabby, brown tabby, blue tabby, cream tabby, cameo tabby, tabby with white, patched tabby with white, tortoiseshell, tortoiseshell with white, calico, dilute calico, blue-cream, blue-cream with white, bi-color, chinchilla silver, shaded silver, shell cameo (red chinchilla), shaded cameo (red shaded), black smoke, blue smoke, cameo smoke (red smoke), blue-cream smoke, and tortie smoke.

EYE COLOR: Eye color should be shades of green, gold, or copper, though white cats may also be either blue or odd-eyed. There is no relationship between eye color and coat color.

Main Coon Cat allowable outcross breeds: None.

MANX

AUTHOR'S NOTE: The Manx is an energetic cat with a distinctive personality that is born out of its great intelligence. It is extremely playful, stubborn, and a bit of a troublemaker. No empty box, bag, or bowl is safe from its four-legged jump. These cats from the Isle of Man in the Irish Sea have no tails, although they can actually have three varieties of tail—the rumpy, no tail at all; stumpy, a tail stump of one to five inches; and the longie, the presence of a complete tail. Only the tailless Manx, however, is accepted for show. The tailed cats are important because when rumpies are bred together for three generations, the kittens do not survive. Manx are great mousers and some even like to swim.

CFA Show Standards

POINT SCORE

HEAD and EARS	25
EYES	5
BODY	25
TAILLESSNESS	15
LEGS and FEET	15
COAT	10
COLOR and MARKINGS	5

GENERAL: The overall impression of the Manx cat is that of roundness—round head with firm, round muzzle and prominent cheeks; broad chest; substantial short front legs; short back that arches from shoulders to a round rump; great depth of flank; and rounded, muscular thighs. The heavy, glossy double coat accentuates the round appearance. With regard to condition, the Manx presented in the show ring should evidence a healthy physical appearance, feeling firm and muscular, neither too fat nor too lean. The Manx should be alert, clear of eye, with a glistening, clean coat.

HEAD and EARS: Round head with prominent cheeks and a jowly appearance. Head is slightly longer than it is broad. Moderately rounded forehead, pronounced cheekbones, and jowliness (jowliness more evident in adult males) enhance the round appearance. Definite whisker break, with large, round whisker pads. In profile there is a gentle nose dip. Well-developed muzzle, slightly longer than broad, with a strong chin. Short, thick neck. Ears wide at the base, tapering gradually to a rounded tip, with sparse interior furnishings. Medium in size in proportion to the head, widely spaced and set slightly outward. When viewed from behind, the ear set resembles the rocker on a cradle.

EYES: Large, round, and full. Set at a slight angle toward the nose (outer corners slightly higher than inner corners). Ideal eye color conforms to requirements of coat color.

BODY: Solidly muscled, compact, and well-balanced, medium in size, with sturdy bone structure. The Manx is stout in appearance, with broad chest and well-sprung ribs; surprisingly heavy when lifted. The constant repetition of curves and circles gives the Manx the appearance of great substance and durability, a cat that is powerful without the slightest hint of coarseness. Males may be somewhat larger than females.

Flank (fleshy area of the side, between the ribs and hip) has greater depth than in other breeds, causing considerable depth to the body when viewed from the side.

The short back forms a smooth, continuous arch from shoulders to rump, curving at the rump to form the desirable round look. Shortness of back is unique to the Manx, but is in proportion to the entire cat and may be somewhat longer in the male.

TAILLESSNESS: Absolute in the perfect specimen, with a decided hollow at the end of the backbone where, in the tailed cat, a tail would begin. A rise of the bones at the end of the spine is allowed and should not be penalized unless it is such that it stops the judge's hand, thereby spoiling the tailless appearance of the cat. The rump is extremely broad and round.

LEGS and FEET: Heavily boned, forelegs short and set well apart to emphasize the broad, deep chest. Hind legs much longer than forelegs, with heavy, muscular thighs and substantial lower legs. Longer hind legs cause the rump to be considerably higher than the shoulders. Hind legs are straight when viewed from behind. Paws are neat and round, with five toes in front and four behind.

COAT: Double coat is short and dense, with a well-padded quality due to the longer, open outer coat and the close, cottony undercoat. Texture of outer guard hairs is somewhat hard; appearance is glossy. Coat may be thicker during cooler months of the year.

TRANSFER TO AOV: Definite, visible tail joint. Long, silky coat.

SEVERELY PENALIZE: If the judge is unable to make the cat stand or walk properly.

DISQUALIFY: Evidence of poor physical condition; incorrect number of toes; evidence of hybridization.

MANX COLORS

White, black, blue, red, cream, chinchilla silver, shaded silver, black smoke, blue smoke, classic tabby pattern, mackerel tabby pattern, patched tabby pattern, brown patched tabby, blue patched tabby, silver patched tabby, silver tabby, red tabby, brown tabby, blue tabby, cream tabby, tortoiseshell, calico, dilute calico, blue-cream, and bi-color.

OMC (Other Manx Colors): Any other color or pattern with the exception of those showing hybridization resulting in the colors chocolate, lavender, the Himalayan pattern, or these in combination with white. **Eye Color**—Appropriate to the predominant color of the cat.

Manx allowable outcross breeds: None.

NORWEGIAN FOREST CAT

AUTHOR'S NOTE: References to the "Norsk Skogkatt" have appeared in Scandinavian poetry, legends, and writings for hundreds of years. It was recognized and shown in Oslow long before World War II, but has only recently been accepted in the CFA where it is currently recognized on a provisional basis. Although similar in appearance to the Maine Coon Cat, the Norwegian Forest Cat is a separate breed. Its back legs are longer than the front legs so that the rump is higher than its shoulders. This clearly distinguishes it from the Maine Coon Cat. It is an independent cat that likes open spaces. Although it accepts domestic life it prefers living in a house that offers it a certain amount of freedom. The Norwegian Forest Cat likes human company but is cautious with strangers. It is an intelligent, fine feline hunter.

CFA Show Standards
(Provisional Standard)

POINT SCORE

HEAD (50)

Nose profile 10

Muzzle 10

Ears 10

Eye shape 5

Eye set 5

Neck 5

Chin 5

BODY (30)

Torso 10

Legs and Feet 10

Boning 5

Tail 5

COAT LENGTH/TEXTURE 5

COLOR/PATTERN 5

CONDITION 5

BALANCE 5

GENERAL: These are very slow-maturing cats, not reaching their full growth until approximately five years of age. At about eight to twelve months of age the development of the skull may cause the eyes to appear too round; this can be forgiven, but not much beyond that age.

HEAD: Front view is a large equilateral triangle measured from cleft of upper lip where it meets lower lip to tip of ear to tip of other ear and back to lip. A second equilateral triangle is measured from cleft of upper lip where it meets lower lip to outer base of ear to outer base of other ear and back to lip. Flat frontal skull. Gently rounded top and rear of skull. Head should not be round or small or long.

NOSE: In profile, straight from tip of nose to just above eyes.

CHIN: Firm in profile. A straight line from nose tip to lower chin line.

MUZZLE: Part of the straight line extending toward the base of ear without pronounced whisker pads and without pinch.

EARS: Slightly taller than width of lower ear opening. Set more to side than on top. Part of the larger equilateral triangle. Furnishings that extend beyond outer edge of ear desired. Lynx tips are desirable but not required.

EYE SHAPE and SET: Almond shape with inner edge rounded. Open and moderately large. On an angle with outer edge tilted toward the lower base of outer ear. Approximately one eye length between eyes.

BODY: Solidly muscled and well-balanced; medium in size, neither long nor cobby. Broad chested with a sturdy bone structure. When measured from the nape of the neck to top of front foot then to rear of back foot, it should be approximately an equal distance. The neck is well developed and relatively short.

LEGS and FEET: Moderately heavily boned. Front feet toe out. Well muscled with good depth of flank. Back legs longer than front so rump is higher than shoulders. Foot feathers desired.

TAIL: Bony part equal in measurement to shoulder. Broader at base and tapering somewhat. Guard hairs desired.

COAT: Double, long guard hairs desired. Long all over body and tail except at back of neck. Full frontal bib, mutton chops and britches highly desirable. May be shorter and less dense in warmer half of year. Texture is relatively silky with multi-colored hairs somewhat firmer than solid hairs. Undercoat and belly hair is of softer and finer texture than guard hairs.

PATTERNS: Every color and pattern is allowable with the exception of those showing hybridization resulting in the colors chocolate, lavender/lilac, the Himalayan pattern, or these combinations with white.

DISQUALIFY: Severe break in nose, square muzzle, whisker pinch, long rectangular body, cobby body.

EYE COLOR: Eye color should be shades of green, gold, or green-gold. White cats may have blue or odd eyes.

NOSE LEATHER and PAW PADS: Any color or combination of colors, not necessarily related to coat color except where so noted. Cats with white on feet may have pink paw pads or they may be bi- or multi-colored.

BUTTONS and LOCKETS: Allowable on any color and/or pattern. Cats with no more than two white spots, whether buttons or lockets, shall be judged as the color of their basic color/pattern. Cats with more than two white spots, whether buttons or lockets, shall be judged as a bi-color, parti-color or "and white," whichever is appropriate.

COAT COLORS: White, black, blue, red, cream, chinchilla silver, shaded silver, chinchilla golden, shaded golden, shell cameo, shaded cameo, shell tortoiseshell, shaded tortoiseshell, black smoke, blue smoke, cream smoke, cameo smoke (red smoke), smoke tortoiseshell, blue-cream smoke, classic tabby pattern, mackerel tabby pattern, patched tabby pattern, spotted tabby pattern, ticked tabby pattern, brown patched tabby, blue patched tabby, silver patched tabby, silver tabby, red tabby, brown tabby, blue tabby, cream tabby, cameo tabby, tortoiseshell, calico, dilute calico, blue-cream, bi-color, van bi-color, van calico, van dilute calico, tabby and white, smoke/shaded/shell and white, tortoiseshell and white, blue-cream and white.

ANY OTHER NFC COLORS: Any other color or pattern with the exception of those showing hybridization resulting in the colors chocolate, lavender/lilac, the Himalayan pattern, or these combinations with white.

Norwegian Forest Cat allowable outcross breeds: None.

OCICAT

AUTHOR'S NOTE: The Ocicat, more than any other domestic cat, resembles its larger, wilder cousins. Its spotted coat suggests a similarity to the ocelot, a spotted leopardlike cat native to the southwestern United States. Despite the resemblance, the Ocicat is far from wild or dangerous. It is friendly and gentle, like all domesticated cats. The Ocicat's primary activity is napping and "talking" to its family. This hybrid breed was created by crossing Siamese and Abyssinians. The current Ocicat is a large, well-spotted, agouti cat (each hair has bands of color) of moderate body type.

CFA Show Standards

POINT SCORE

HEAD (25)
> Skull. 5
> Muzzle. 10
> Ears. 5
> Eyes. 5

BODY (25)
> Size. 5
> Torso. 10
> Legs and feet. 5
> Tail. 5

COAT and COLOR (25)
> Texture. 5
> Coat Color. 5
> Contrast. 10
> Eye Color. 5

PATTERN. 25

GENERAL: The Ocicat is a medium to large, well-spotted agouti cat of moderate type. It displays the look of an athletic animal: well muscled and solid, graceful and lithe, yet with a fullness of body and chest. It is alert to its surroundings and shows great vitality. The Ocicat is found in many colors, with darker spots appearing on a lighter background. Each hair (except on the tip of tail) has several bands of color. It is where these bands fall together that a thumbprint-shaped spot is formed. This powerful, athletic, yet graceful, spotted cat is particularly noted for its "wild" appearance.

HEAD: The skull is a modified wedge showing a slight curve from muzzle to cheek, with a visible, but gentle, rise from the bridge of the nose to the brow. The muzzle is broad and well defined, with a suggestion of squareness, and in profile shows good length. The chin is strong and the jaw firm, with a proper bite. The moderate whisker pinch is not too severe. The head is carried gracefully on an arching neck. An allowance is made for jowls on mature males.

EARS: Alert, moderately large, and set so as to corner the upper, outside dimensions of the head. If an imaginary horizontal line is drawn across the brow, the ears should be set at a forty-five degree angle, i.e. neither too high nor too low. When they occur, ear tufts extending vertically from the tips of the ears are a bonus.

EYES: Large, almond-shaped, and angling slightly upward toward the ears, with more than the length of an eye between the eyes.

SIZE: Medium to large. The Ocicat should have a surprising weight for its size. It should be noted that females are generally smaller than males. The overall structure and quality of this cat should be of greater consideration than mere size alone.

TORSO: Solid, rather long-bodied, with depth and fullness, but never coarse. Substantial bone and muscle development, yet with an athletic appearance. There should be some depth of chest, with ribs slightly sprung, the back is level to slightly higher in the rear, and the flank reasonably level. Preference is given to the athletic, powerful, and lithe, and objection taken to the bulky or coarse.

LEGS and FEET: Legs should be of good substance and well muscled, medium-long, powerful, and in good proportion to the body. Feet should be oval and compact, with five toes in front and four in back, with size in proportion to legs.

TAIL: Fairly long, medium-slim, with only a slight taper and with a dark tip.

COAT TEXTURE: Short, smooth, and satiny in texture, with a lustrous sheen. Tight, close-lying, and sleek, yet long enough to accommodate the necessary bands of color. There should be no suggestion of woolliness.

TICKING: All hairs except the tip of the tail are banded. Within the markings, hairs are tipped with a darker color, while hairs in the ground color are tipped with a lighter color.

COAT COLOR: All colors should be clear and pleasing. The lightest color is usually found on the face, around the eyes, and on the chin and lower jaw. The darkest color is found on the tip of the tail. Contrast is scored separately.

CONTRAST: Distinctive markings should be clearly seen from any orientation. Those on the face, legs, and tail may be darker than those on the torso. Ground color may be darker on the saddle and lighter on the underside, chin, and lower jaw. Penalties should be given if spotting is faint or blurred, though it must be remembered that pale colors will show less contrast than darker ones.

EYE COLOR: All eye colors except blue are allowed. There is no correspondence between eye color and coat color. Depth of color is preferred.

PATTERN: There is an intricate tabby "M" on the forehead, with markings extending up over the head, between the ears, and breaking into small spots on the lower neck and shoulders. "Mascara" markings are found around the eyes and on cheeks. Rows of round spots run along the spine, from shoulder blades to tail. The tail has horizontal brush strokes down the top, ideally alternating with spots, and a dark tip. Spots are scattered across the shoulders and hindquarters, extending as far as possible down the legs. There are broken bracelets on the lower legs and broken necklaces at the throat—the more broken the better. Large, well-scattered, thumbprint-shaped spots appear on the sides of the torso, with a subtle suggestion of a classic tabby pattern—a spot circled by spots in place of the bull's-eye. The belly is also well spotted. The eyes are rimmed with the darkest coat color and surrounded by the lightest color. Penalties should be given for elongated spots following a mackerel pattern.

DISQUALIFY: White locket or spotting, or white anywhere

other than around eyes, nostrils, chin, and upper throat (except white agouti ground in silvered colors). Kinked or otherwise deformed tail. Blue eyes. Incorrect number of toes. Due to the spotted, patched tabby (torbie) cats resulting from the sex-linked O gene, no reds, creams, or torbies are allowed. Very rufous cinnamons and fawns may resemble red or cream, but never produce female torbies.

OCICAT COLORS

Tawny, chocolate, cinnamon, blue, lavender, fawn, silver, chocolate silver, cinnamon silver, blue silver, lavender silver, and fawn silver.

Ocicat allowable outcross breeds: Abyssinian for litters born before 1/1/95.

ORIENTAL SHORTHAIR

AUTHOR'S NOTE: The personality of the Oriental Short-hair is similar to that of the Siamese, including its very talkative nature. It is an outgoing cat, quite assertive, and knows how to get what it wants, which is usually total attention from its family. It was created by crossing the Siamese with shorthair solid colors and Russian Blues. It is a Siamese cat that is "self-colored," which means solid-colored with no point-color contrast. The most popular colors are those of the Siamese points, such as chocolate or lilac. The Oriental Shorthair is a by-product of the efforts to create a solid-colored brown Siamese, which ultimately became the Havana Brown. The breed was accepted by CFA for registration and showing in 1972 and entered championship competition in 1977. The standards for the Oriental Shorthair and the Siamese are almost identical, except for color and coat pattern.

CFA Show Standards

POINT SCORE

HEAD (20)
    Long, flat profile 6
    Wedge, fine muzzle, size 5

GENERAL: The ideal Oriental Shorthair is a svelte cat with long, tapering lines, very lithe but muscular. Excellent physical condition. Eyes clear. Strong and lithe, neither bony nor flabby. Not fat.

HEAD: Long, tapering wedge, in good proportion to body. The total wedge starts at the nose and flares out in straight lines to the tips of the ears, forming a triangle, with no break at the whiskers. No less than the width of an eye between the eyes. When the whiskers are smoothed back, the underlying bone structure is apparent. Allowance must be made for jowls in the stud cat.

SKULL: Flat. In profile, a long, straight line is seen from the top of the head to the tip of the nose. No bulge over eyes. No dip in nose.

NOSE: Long and straight. A continuation of the forehead, with no break.

MUZZLE: Fine, wedge-shaped.

CHIN and JAW: Medium size. Tip of chin lines up with tip of nose in the same vertical plane. Neither receding nor excessively massive.

EARS: Strikingly large, pointed, wide at the base, continuing the lines of the wedge.

EYES: Almond shaped, medium size. Neither protruding nor recessed. Slanted toward the nose in harmony with lines of wedge and ears. Uncrossed.

BODY: Long and svelte. A distinctive combination of fine bones and firm muscles. Shoulders and hips continue the same sleek lines of tubular body. Hips never wider than shoulders. Abdomen tight. Males may be somewhat larger than females.

NECK: Long and slender.

LEGS: Long and slim. Hind legs higher than front. In good proportion to body.

PAWS: Dainty, small and oval. Toes: five in front and four behind.

TAIL: Long, thin at the base, and tapered to a fine point.

COAT: Short, fine-textured, glossy, lying close to body.

COAT COLOR: The Oriental Shorthair's reason for being is the coat color, whether it is solid or tabby patterned. In the solid-color cat, the coat color should be of uniform density and color from the tip to the root of each hair and from the nose to the tail. The full coat-color score (20) should be used to assess the quality and the correctness of the color. In the tabby-patterned cat, the quality of the pattern is an essential part of the cat. The pattern should match the description for the particular pattern and be well defined. The pattern should be viewed while the cat is in a natural standing position. Ten points are allotted to the correctness of the color; it matches the color description. The division of points for coat color applies only to the Tabby Colors Class.

PENALIZE: Crossed eyes. Palpable and/or visible protrusion of the cartilage at the end of the sternum.

DISQUALIFY: Any evidence of illness or poor health. Weak hind legs. Mouth breathing due to nasal obstruction or poor occlusion. Emaciation. Visible kink. Miniaturization. Lockets and buttons. Incorrect number of toes.

EYE COLOR: Green. White Orientals may have blue, green, or odd-eyed eye color.

ORIENTAL SHORTHAIR COLORS

Blue, chestnut, cinnamon, cream, ebony, fawn, lavender, red, white, blue-cream silver, blue silver, cameo, dilute cameo (cream silver), chestnut silver, chestnut-tortie silver, cinnamon silver, cinnamon-tortie silver, ebony silver, fawn silver, lavender-cream silver, lavender silver, tortoiseshell silver, blue smoke, cameo smoke (red smoke), chestnut smoke, cinnamon smoke, dilute cameo smoke, ebony smoke, fawn smoke, lavender smoke, parti-color smoke, classic tabby pattern, mackerel tabby pattern, spotted tabby pattern, ticked tabby pattern, patched tabby pattern, blue silver tabby, blue tabby, cameo tabby, dilute cameo tabby, cinnamon silver tabby, cinnamon tabby, chestnut silver tabby, chestnut tabby, cream tabby, ebony tabby, fawn tabby, fawn silver tabby, lavender silver tabby, lavender tabby, red tabby, silver tabby, blue-cream, cinnamon tortoiseshell, chestnut tortoiseshell, fawn-cream, lavender-cream, and ebony tortoiseshell.

Oriental Shorthair allowable outcross breeds: Siamese or Colorpoint.

PERSIAN

AUTHOR'S NOTE: Persians are among the most beautiful cats in the world. They exude great dignity. Few breeds are as popular or as successful. Their popularity can be attributed to their luxuriously overflowing, longhair coats and to their quiet poise. However, no matter how docile they appear to be, they constantly demand the attention of their families and can be quite insistent about it. And there is nothing dainty about a Persian. Under all that fluffy coat is a stocky, heavy body supported by legs that are short, thick, and strong. They are not active cats and sit quietly, staring at the passing world, when they are not sleeping. Their profuse coats require a great deal of grooming fuss and attention. No one knows where the Persian came from. The origin of this breed remains an unsolved mystery in the cat world. Many believe the birthplace of this natural breed is somewhere in Persia (Iran) or Turkey, but the exact location is unknown. Although Persians are ancient, they can also be classified as a modern breed because they are the result of highly selective breeding programs begun in the late nineteenth century.

CFA Show Standards

POINT SCORE

Head (including size and shape of eyes, ear shape and
set) 30
Type (including shape, size, bone, and length of tail) . . 20
Coat 10
Balance 5
Refinement 5
Color 20
Eye color 10

In all tabby varieties, the 20 points for color are to be
divided 10 for markings and 10 for color. In all "with
white" varieties (calico, dilute calico, bi-color, van bi-color,
van calico, van dilute calico, and tabby and white), the 20
points for color are to be divided 10 for "with white"
pattern and 10 for color.

GENERAL: The ideal Persian should present an impression
of a heavily boned, well-balanced cat with a sweet expression
and soft, round lines. The large, round eyes set wide apart in a
large, round head contribute to the overall look and expression.
The long, thick coat softens the lines of the cat and accentuates
the roundness in appearance.

HEAD: Round and massive, with great breadth of skull.
Round face with round underlying bone structure. Well set on
a short, thick neck.

NOSE: Short, snub, and broad. With "break."

CHEEKS: Full.

JAWS: Broad and powerful.

CHIN: Full, well-developed, and firmly rounded, reflecting
a proper bite.

EARS: Small, round-tipped, tilted forward, and not unduly
open at the base. Set far apart, and low on the head, fitting into
(without distorting) the rounded contour of the head.

EYES: Brilliant in color, large, round, and full. Set level and
far apart, giving a sweet expression to the face.

BODY: Of cobby type, low on the legs, broad and deep through the chest, equally massive across the shoulders and rump, with a well-rounded midsection and level back. Good muscle tone, with no evidence of obesity. Large or medium in size. Quality the determining consideration rather than size.

LEGS: Short, thick, and strong. Forelegs straight.

PAWS: Large, round, and firm. Toes carried close, five in front and four behind.

TAIL: Short, but in proportion to body length. Carried without a curve and at an angle lower than the back.

COAT: Long and thick, standing off from the body. Of fine texture, glossy and full of life. Long all over the body, including the shoulders. The ruff immense and continuing in a deep frill between the front legs. Ear and toe tufts long. Brush very full.

DISQUALIFY: Locket or button. Kinked or abnormal tail. Incorrect number of toes. Any apparent weakness in the hindquarters. Any apparent deformity of the spine. Deformity of the skull resulting in an asymmetrical face and/or head. Crossed eyes. For pointed cats, also disqualify for white toes, eye color other than blue.*

PERSIAN COLORS

White, black, blue, red, cream, chocolate, lilac, chinchilla silver, shaded silver, chinchilla golden, shaded golden, shell cameo (red chinchilla), shaded cameo (red shaded), shell tortoiseshell, shaded tortoiseshell, black smoke, blue smoke, cameo smoke (red smoke), smoke tortoiseshell, blue-cream smoke, classic tabby pattern, mackerel tabby pattern, patched tabby pattern, brown patched tabby, blue patched tabby, silver patched tabby, silver tabby, red tabby, brown tabby, blue tabby, cream tabby, cameo tabby, tortoiseshell, calico, dilute calico, blue-cream, bi-color, van bi-color, van calico, van dilute calico, tabby and white, peke-face red and peke-face red tabby, seal point, chocolate point, blue point, lilac point, flame (red)

*The above-listed disqualifications apply to all Persian cats.

point, cream point, tortie point, chocolate-tortie point, blue-cream point, lilac-cream point, seal lynx point, blue lynx point, tortie lynx point, and blue-cream lynx point.

Persian allowable outcross breeds: None.

RUSSIAN BLUE

AUTHOR'S NOTE: The Russian Blue is an elegant cat that is ideally suited to a quiet environment. It is gentle and self-composed most of the time, except when it is in one of its demanding phases. These cats are hardly vocal at all, affectionate with their families but hesitant with visitors. The most striking feature of this breed is its plush but fine coat. In the cat world, "blue" means a rich gray tinted with a suggestion of blue. In the case of the Russian Blue, the undercoat of this warm, sumptuous-looking cat is "blue" and the outer coat is tipped with silver. Add to this effect the lavender-pink color of the paw pads and the vivid green eyes, and you have a dazzlingly beautiful cat. Russian Blues originated in Archangel, Northern Russia. It's a cold, arctic climate, and a warm double coat is a necessity for any animal living there. These Russians came to the North American shores at the turn of the century, via England.

CFA Show Standards

POINT SCORE

HEAD and NECK	20
BODY TYPE	20
EYE SHAPE	5
EARS	5
COAT	20
COLOR	20
EYE COLOR	10

GENERAL: The good show specimen has good physical condition, is firm in muscle tone, and alert.

HEAD: Smooth, medium wedge, neither long and tapering

nor short and massive. Muzzle is blunt, and part of the total wedge, without exaggerated pinch or whisker break. Top of skull long and flat in profile, gently descending to slightly above the eyes, and continuing, at a slight downward angle, in a straight line to the tip of the nose. No nose break or stop. Length of top-head should be greater than length of nose. The face is broad across the eyes due to wide eye-set and thick fur.

MUZZLE: Smooth, flowing wedge without prominent whisker pads or whisker pinches.

EARS: Rather large and wide at the base. Tips more pointed than rounded. The skin of the ears is thin and translucent, with little inside furnishing. The outside of the ear is scantily covered with short, very fine hair, with leather showing through. Set far apart, as much on the side as on the top of the head.

EYES: Set wide apart. Aperture rounded in shape.

NECK: Long and slender, but appearing short due to thick fur and high placement of shoulder blades.

NOSE: Medium in length.

CHIN: Perpendicular with the end of the nose and with level under-chin. Neither receding nor excessively massive.

BODY: Fine-boned, long, firm, and muscular; lithe and graceful in outline and carriage without being tubular in appearance.

LEGS: Long and fine-boned.

PAWS: Small, slightly rounded. Toes: five in front and four behind.

TAIL: Long, but in proportion to the body. Tapering from a moderately thick base.

COAT: Short, dense, fine, and plush. Double coat stands out from body due to density. It has a distinct soft and silky feel.

DISQUALIFY: Kinked or abnormal tail. Locket or button. Incorrect number of toes.

RUSSIAN BLUE COLOR

Even, bright blue throughout. Lighter shades of blue preferred. Guard hairs distinctly silver-tipped, giving the cat a silvery sheen or lustrous appearance. A definite contrast should be noted between ground color and tipping. Free from tabby markings. **Nose leather**—Slate gray. **Paw pads**—Lavender-pink or mauve. **Eye color**—Vivid green.

Russian Blue allowable outcross breeds: None.

SCOTTISH FOLD

AUTHOR'S NOTE: This cat is called the Scottish Fold because of its unique ears, the top halves of which fold forward, giving it a quizzical look. The breed is considered a mutation, with an unusual recessive gene that causes the ears to fold down in the middle. Other outstanding features are its eyes. These cats are like large drops of sweet syrup that stare out at you with affection. They are good-natured cats, with a warm, friendly spirit and a live-and-let-live attitude. They hardly speak and may stay in one resting place for the longest time. Because they seem to appreciate their homes, their owners tend to give them anything they want. These are among the most endearing creatures on Earth. The Scottish Fold appeared in Perthshire, Scotland, in the 1960s. It is characterized by a softly rounded head; short, muscular body; and thick, sometimes marbled, shorthaired coat. Everything about this cat is round—its head, eyes, even its body.

CFA Show Standards

POINT SCORE

HEAD (55)
    Ears 25
    Head shape, muzzle, neck, chin, profile 15
    Eyes 15
BODY (40)
    Body structure of torso, legs and paws 10
    Tail 20
    Coat 10
COLOR (5)
    Color of coat and eyes 5

GENERAL: The Scottish Fold cat occurred as a spontaneous mutation in farm cats in Scotland. The breed has been established by crosses to British Shorthair and domestic cats in Scotland and England. In America, the outcross is the American and British Shorthair. All bona fide Scottish Fold cats trace their pedigree to Susie, the first fold-ear cat, discovered by the founders of the breed, William and Mary Ross.

HEAD: Well rounded with a firm chin and jaw. Muzzle to have well-rounded whisker pads. Head should blend into a short neck. Prominent cheeks, with a jowly appearance in males.

EYES: Wide open, with a sweet expression. Large, well rounded, and separated by a broad nose. Eye color to correspond with coat color. Blue-eyed and odd-eyed are allowed for white and white-dominated coat patterns, e.g., all van patterns.

NOSE: Nose to be short with a gentle curve. A brief stop is permitted, but a definite nose break considered a fault. Profile is moderate in appearance.

EARS: Fold forward and downward. Small, the smaller, tightly folded ear preferred over a loose fold and large ear. The ears should be set in a cap-like fashion to expose a rounded cranium. Ear tips to be rounded.

BODY: Medium, rounded, and even from shoulder to pelvic girdle. The cat should stand firm on a well-padded body. There must be no hint of thickness or lack of mobility in the cat due to short, coarse legs. Toes to be neat and well rounded, with five in front and four behind. Overall appearance is that of a well-founded cat with medium bone; fault cats obviously lacking in type. Females may be slightly smaller.

TAIL: Tail should be medium to long but in proportion to the body. Tail should be flexible and tapering. Longer, tapering tail preferred.

COAT: Dense, plush, medium-short, soft in texture, full of life. Standing out from body due to density; not flat or close-lying. Coat texture may vary due to color and/or region or seasonal changes.

DISQUALIFY: Kinked tail. Tail that is foreshortened. Tail

that is lacking in flexibility due to abnormally thick vertebrae. Incorrect number of toes. Any evidence of illness or poor health.

SCOTTISH FOLD COLORS

White, black, blue, red, cream, chinchilla silver, shaded silver, shell cameo (red chinchilla), shaded cameo (red shaded), black smoke, blue smoke, cameo smoke (red smoke), classic tabby pattern, mackerel tabby pattern, patched tabby pattern, spotted tabby pattern, silver tabby, red tabby, brown tabby, blue tabby, cream tabby, cameo tabby, tortoiseshell, calico, dilute calico, blue-cream, bi-color.

OSFC (Other Scottish Fold Colors): Any other color or pattern with the exception of those showing evidence of hybridization resulting in the colors chocolate, lavender, the Himalayan pattern, or these combinations with white. **Eye color**—Appropriate to the dominant color of the cat.

Scottish Fold allowable outcross breeds: British Shorthair, American Shorthair.

SIAMESE

AUTHOR'S NOTE: The mind of the Siamese approaches cat genius. It is an intelligent animal with an affectionate nature and a strong desire to be a lively, active member of the family it lives with. It is said of the Siamese that its behavior is fairly close to that of the dog in its desire to please and relate to humans. It has a natural inclination to fetch, bow, and learn any trick you are capable of teaching it. Its voice is unequaled on the face of the earth, and it will talk and talk and talk, especially about dinner, and your lap to settle into. Although the breed was once stocky and round-headed, it is now bred and shown with a sleek, tubular-shaped body, fine-boned, and a head that comes to a tapered wedge, punctuated by large, pointed ears. Its almond-shaped eyes must be uncrossed, and its nose should be perfectly in line with the contours of its face. The Siamese is a natural, ancient breed that is often used in crossbreeding experiments, which have resulted in creating many of today's popular breeds, such as the Balinese, Havana Brown, Himalayan, and Tonkinese. The outstanding physical feature of this outstanding cat is its contrasting color pattern called "colorpoint." "Point" (meaning darker) refers to the facial mask, ears, legs, and tail, which are a rich dark color in contrast to the rest of the body. In North America, only the four basic colors are considered Siamese. They are Seal point, chocolate point, blue point, and lilac point. See "Siamese Colors."

CFA Show Standards

POINT SCORE

HEAD (20)
 Long, flat profile 6
 Wedge, fine muzzle, size 5
 Ears 4
 Chin 3
 Width between eyes 2
EYES (10)
 Shape, size, slant, and placement 10
BODY (30)
 Structure and size, including Neck 12
 Muscle tone 10
 Legs and Feet 5
 Tail 3
COAT 10
COLOR (30)
 Body color 10
 Point color (matching points of dense color, proper
   foot pads and nose leather) 10
 Eye color 10

GENERAL: The ideal Siamese is a medium-sized, svelte, refined cat with long, tapering lines, very lithe but muscular. Males may be proportionately larger.

HEAD: Long, tapering wedge. Medium in size body. The

total wedge starts at the nose and flares out in straight lines to the tips of the ears, forming a triangle, with no break at the whiskers. No less than the width of an eye between the eyes. When the whiskers are smoothed back, the underlying bone structure is apparent. Allowance must be made for jowls in the stud cat.

SKULL: Flat. In profile, a long, straight line is seen from the top of the head to the tip of the nose. No bulge over eyes. No dip in nose.

EARS: Strikingly large, pointed, wide at base; continuing the lines of the wedge.

EYES: Almond-shaped. Medium size. Neither protruding nor recessed. Slanted toward the nose, in harmony with lines of wedge and ears. Uncrossed.

NOSE: Long and straight. A continuation of the forehead, with no break.

MUZZLE: Fine, wedge-shaped.

CHIN and JAW: Medium size. Tip of chin lines up with tip of nose in the same vertical plane. Neither receding nor excessively massive.

BODY: Medium size. Graceful, long, and svelte. A distinctive combination of fine bones and firm muscles. Shoulders and hips continue same sleek lines of tubular body. Hips never wider than shoulders. Abdomen tight.

NECK: Long and slender.

LEGS: Long and slim. Hind legs higher than front. In good proportion to body.

PAWS: Dainty, small, and oval. Toes: five in front and four behind.

TAIL: Long, thin, tapering to a fine point.

COAT: Short, fine-textured, glossy. Lying close to body.

CONDITION: Excellent physical condition. Eyes clear. Muscular, strong, and lithe. Neither flabby nor bony. Not fat.

COLOR: Body—Even, with subtle shading when allowed. Allowance should be made for darker color in older cats, as Siamese generally darken with age, but there must be definite contrast between body color and points. Points—Mask, ears, legs, feet, tail dense and clearly defined. All of the same shade. Mask covers entire face, including whisker pads, and is connected to ears by tracings. Mask should not extend over the top of the head. No ticking or white hairs in points.

PENALIZE: Improper (i.e., off-color or spotted) nose leather or paw pads. Soft or mushy body.

DISQUALIFY: Any evidence of illness or poor health. Weak hind legs. Mouth breathing due to nasal obstruction or poor occlusion. Emaciation. Visible kink. Eyes other than blue. White toes and/or feet. Incorrect number of toes. Malocclusion resulting in either undershot or overshot chin.

SIAMESE COLORS

SEAL POINT: Body even pale fawn to cream, warm in tone, shading gradually into lighter color on the stomach and chest. Points deep seal brown. **Nose leather and paw pads**—Same color as points. **Eye color**—Deep, vivid blue.

CHOCOLATE POINT: Body ivory with no shading. Points milk-chocolate color, warm in tone. **Nose leather and paw pads**—Cinnamon-pink. **Eye color**—Deep, vivid blue.

BLUE POINT: Body bluish white, cold in tone, shading gradually to white on stomach and chest. Points deep blue. **Nose leather and paw pads**—Slate colored. **Eye color**—Deep, vivid blue.

LILAC POINT: Body glacial white with no shading. Points frosty gray with pinkish tone. **Nose leather and paw pads**—Lavender-pink. **Eye color**—Deep, vivid blue.

Siamese allowable outcross breeds: None.

SINGAPURA

AUTHOR'S NOTE: This rare and unusual cat was first accepted by CFA for registration in 1982, and for championship competition in 1988. Its personality includes extreme curiosity blended with boldness. The Singapura will hop into any situation and roam around kitchen counters, closets, and every nook and cranny of your home. It is a friendly cat that fearlessly approaches all visitors and invites them to play.

These are "people" cats and develop strong attachments to their families. The Singapura is a natural breed, native to Southeast Asia and named after the great island of Singapore, at the south end of the Malay Peninsula. The breed was found on the streets of the city of Singapore by several Americans living there and was imported to the United States in 1975. An additional import entered the U.S. in 1980. The Singapura is a small cat bearing a ticked coat pattern similar to that of the Abyssinian. Both breeds resemble miniature cougars. All other characteristics of the Singapura, however, are different from those of the Abyssinian. Its coat, with reddish-brown color and two bands of dark ticking separated by light bands, makes it a very attractive cat.

CFA Show Standards

POINT SCORE

HEAD (25)
Ears 10
Head Shape 4
Width at Eye 4
Muzzle Shape 4
Profile 3
EYES (10)
Size and Placement 6
Shape 3
Color 1
BODY, LEGS and TAIL (20)
Neck 3
Proportion 10
Legs and Feet 5
Tail 2
COAT 15
COLOR 15
MARKINGS 15

GENERAL: The appearance of an alert, healthy, small-to-medium-size, muscular-bodied cat with noticeably large eyes and ears. Cat to have the illusion of refined, delicate coloring.

HEAD: Skull rounded, with rounded width at the outer eye narrowing to a definite whisker break and a medium-short, broad muzzle with a blunt nose. In profile, a rounded skull with a very slight stop well below eye level. Straight line nose to chin. Chin well developed.

EARS: Large, slightly pointed, wide open at the base, and possessing a deep cup. Medium-set. Outer lines of the ear to extend upward at an angle slightly wide of parallel. Small ears a serious fault.

EYES: Large, almond-shaped, held wide open but showing slant. Neither protruding nor recessed. Eyes set not less than an eye width apart. Color hazel, green, or yellow, with no other color permitted. Brilliance preferred. Small eyes a serious fault.

BODY: Small-to-medium overall size cat. Moderately stocky and muscular. Body, legs, and floor form a square. Mid-section not tucked but firm.

NECK: Short and thick.

LEGS and FEET: Legs heavy and muscled at the body, tapering to small, short, oval feet.

TAIL: Length to be short of the shoulder when laid along the torso. Tending toward slender but not whippy. Blunt tip.

COAT: Fine, very short, lying very close to the body. Allowance for longer coat in kittens. Springy coat a fault.

MARKINGS: Each hair to have at least two bands of dark ticking separated by light bands. Light next to skin and a dark tip. Dark tail tip, with color extending back toward the body on the upper side. Cat to show some barring on inner front legs and back knee only. Allowance to be made for undeveloped ticking in kittens. Spine line NOT a fault.

PENALIZE: Dark coat coloring next to skin, definite gray tones, barring on outer front legs, necklaces, non-visible tail faults.

DISQUALIFY: White lockets, barring on tail, top of the head unticked, unbroken necklaces or leg bracelets. Very small eyes or ears. Visible tail faults.

SINGAPURA COLOR

COLOR: Color to be dark brown ticking on a warm old-ivory ground color. Muzzle, chin, chest, and stomach to be the color of unbleached muslin. Nose leather pale to dark salmon. Eyeliner, nose outline, lips, whisker apertures, hair between the toes to be dark brown. Foot pads a rosy brown. Salmon tones to the ears and nose bridge NOT a fault. Warm, light shades preferred.

Singapura allowable outcross breeds: None.

SOMALI

AUTHOR'S NOTE: The Somali is like the Abyssinian in every way except for its coat. It has a fine double coat that is of medium length, with a full brush tail giving it an outstanding look and placing it in the longhair category. The Somali personality is also similar to that of the Abyssinian. It is the motorcycle of the cat breeds with its fast starts and speedy runs around the house. These are highly spirited, affectionate, and extremely playful cats. There have been random longhair mutations in Abyssinian litters for years. In the 1970s these handsome rarities were finally bred to create the Somali. They retain all the characteristic Abyssinian traits, such as the agouti coloring (each hair is individually striped with brown or black) and that active, assertive, spirited personality.

CFA Show Standards

POINT SCORE

HEAD (25)
    Skull 6
    Muzzle 6
    Ears 7
    Eye shape 6
BODY (25)
    Torso 10
    Legs and Feet 10
    Tail 5

COAT (25)
    Texture. 10
    Length. 15
COLOR (25)
    Color. 10
    Ticking. 10
    Eye color 5

GENERAL: The overall impression of the Somali is that of a well-proportioned medium-to-large cat, firm muscular development, lithe, showing an alert, lively interest in all surroundings, with an even disposition and easy to handle. The cat is to give the appearance of activity, sound health, and general vigor.

HEAD: A modified, slightly rounded wedge without flat planes; the brow, cheek, and profile lines all showing a gentle contour. A slight rise from the bridge of the nose to the forehead, which should be of good size, with width between the ears flowing into the arched neck without a break.

MUZZLE: Shall follow gentle contours in conformity with the skull, as viewed from the front profile. Chin shall be full, neither undershot nor overshot, having a rounded appearance. The muzzle shall not be sharply pointed, and there shall be no evidence of snippiness, foxiness, or whisker pinch. Allowance to be made for jowls in adult males.

EARS: Large, alert, moderately pointed, broad, and cupped at the base. Ear set on a line toward the rear of the skull. The inner ear shall have horizontal tufts that reach nearly to the other side of the ear; tufts desirable.

EYES: Almond shaped, large, brilliant, and expressive. Skull aperture neither round nor oriental. Eyes accented by dark lid skin encircled by light colored area. Above each a short, dark, vertical pencil stroke with a dark pencil line continuing from the upper lid toward the ear.

BODY: Torso medium long, lithe, and graceful, showing well-developed muscular strength. Rib cage is rounded; back is slightly arched, giving the appearance of a cat about to spring;

flank level, with no tuck up. Conformation strikes a medium between the extremes of cobby and svelte lengthy types.

LEGS and FEET: Legs in proportion to torso; feet oval and compact. When standing, the Somali gives the impression of being nimble and quick. Toes: five in front and four in back.

TAIL: Having a full brush, thick at the base, and slightly tapering. Length in balance with torso.

COAT: Texture very soft to the touch, extremely fine and double coated. The more dense the coat, the better. Length—A medium-length coat, except over shoulders, where a slightly shorter length is permitted. Preference is to be given to a cat with ruff and breeches, giving a full-coated appearance to the cat.

PENALIZE: Color faults—Cold gray or sandy tone to coat color; mottling or speckling on unticked areas. Pattern faults—Necklaces, legs bars, tabby stripes, or bars on body; lack of desired markings on head and tail. Black roots on body.

DISQUALIFY: White locket or groin spot, or white anywhere on body other than on the upper throat, chin, or nostrils. Any skeletal abnormality. Wrong color paw pads or nose leather. Unbroken necklace. Incorrect number of toes. Kinks in tail.

SOMALI COLORS

RUDDY: Overall impression of an orange-brown or ruddy ticked with black. Color has radiant or glowing quality. Darker shading along the spine allowed. Underside of body and inside of legs and chest to be an even ruddy tone, harmonizing with the top coat; without ticking, barring, necklaces, or belly marks. **Nose leather**—Tile red. **Paw pads**—Black or brown, with black between toes and extending upward on rear legs. Off-white on upper throat, lips, and nostrils only. Tail continuing the dark spine line, ending in black at the tip. Complete absence of rings on tail. Preference given to unmarked ruddy color. Ears tipped with black or dark brown. **Eye color**—Gold or green, the more richness and depth of color the better.

RED: Warm, glowing red ticked with chocolate-brown.

Deeper shades of red preferred. Ears and tail tipped with chocolate-brown. **Nose leather**—Rosy pink. **Paw pads**—Pink with chocolate-brown between toes, extending slightly beyond paws. **Eye color**—Gold or green, the more richness and depth the better.

BLUE: Coat warm beige, ticked with various shades of slate blue, the extreme outer tip to be the darkest, with blush beige undercoat. Tail tipped with slate blue. The underside and inside of the legs to be a tint to harmonize with the main color. **Nose leather**—Old rose. **Paw pads**—Mauve, with slate blue between toes, extending slightly beyond the paws. **Eye color**—Gold or green, the more richness and depth of color the better.

FAWN: Coat warm rose-beige, ticked with light cocoa brown, the extreme outer tip to be the darkest, with a blush beige undercoat. Tail tipped with light cocoa brown. The underside and inside of legs to be a tint to harmonize with the main color. **Nose leather**—Salmon. **Paw pads**—Pink, with light cocoa brown between the toes, extending slightly beyond the paws. **Eye color**—Gold or green, the more richness and depth the better.

(PLEASE NOTE: The Somali is extremely slow in showing mature ticking, and allowances should be made for kittens and young cats.)

Somali allowable outcross breeds: Abyssinian.

TONKINESE

AUTHOR'S NOTE: Although the Tonkinese is a close cousin to the Siamese (and the Burmese), it is different in the shape of its body and the color of its coat. Its body represents a balance between the foreign type (tubular-shaped, fine-boned) and the cobby type (deep-chested, large-boned, compact). Unlike the Siamese, the Tonkinese's point color does not contrast sharply with its ground-coat color. The Tonkinese's ground coat is always a dilution (lighter shade) of the same, darker point color. The Tonkinese is a fun-loving cat that is intelligent, affectionate, and full of mischief. It is very playful, too playful

*for some, but adjusts well to a household with children and
other pets.*

CFA Show Standards

POINT SCORE

HEAD (25)
    Profile 8
    Muzzle 6
    Ears 6
    Eye shape and set .5
BODY (30)
    Torso 15
    Legs and Feet 5
    Tail 5
    Muscle tone 5
COAT 10
COLOR (35)
    Body color 15
    Point color 10
    Eye color 10

GENERAL: The Tonkinese cat was originally the result of a
Siamese to Burmese breeding. The ideal Tonkinese is intermediate in type, being neither cobby nor svelte. The Tonkinese
should give the overall impression of an alert, active cat with
good muscular development. The cat should be surprisingly
heavy. While the breed is to be considered medium in size,
balance and proportion are of greater importance.

HEAD and MUZZLE: The head is a modified wedge
somewhat longer than it is wide, with high, gently planed
cheekbones. The muzzle is blunt, as long as it is wide. There is
a slight whisker break, gently curved, following the lines of the
wedge. There is a slight stop at eye level. In profile the tip of
the chin lines with the tip of the nose in the same vertical plane.
There is a gentle rise from the tip of the nose to the stop. There
is a gentle contour, with a slight rise from the nose stop to the
forehead. There is a slight convex curve to the forehead.

EARS: Alert, medium in size. Oval tips, broad at the base. Ears set as much on the sides of the head as on the top. Hair on the ears very short and close-lying. Leather may show through.

EYES: Open almond shape. Slanted along the cheekbones toward the outer edge of the ear. Eyes are proportionate in size to the face.

EYE COLOR: Aqua. A definitive characteristic of the Tonkinese breed, best seen in natural light. Depth, clarity, and brilliance of color preferred.

BODY: Torso medium in length, demonstrating well-developed muscular strength without coarseness. The Tonkinese conformation strikes a midpoint between the extremes of long, svelte body types and cobby, compact body types. Balance and proportion are more important than size alone. The abdomen should be taut, well-muscled, and firm.

LEGS and FEET: Fairly slim, proportionate in length and bone to the body. Hind legs slightly longer than front. Paws more oval than round. Trim. Toes: five in front and four behind.

TAIL: Proportionate in length to body. Tapering.

COAT: Medium-short in length, close-lying, fine, soft, and silky, with a lustrous sheen.

BODY COLOR: The mature specimen should be a rich, even, unmarked color, shading almost imperceptibly to a slightly lighter hue on the underparts. Allowance to be made for lighter body color in young cats. With the dilute colors in particular, development of full body color may take up to sixteen months. Cats do darken with age, but there must be a distinct contrast between body color and points.

POINT COLOR: Mask, ears, feet, and tail all densely marked, but merging gently into body color. Except in kittens, mask and ears should be connected by tracings. Allowance to be made for slight barring in young cats.

PENALIZE: Palpable tail fault. Extreme ranginess or cobbiness. Definite nose break. Round eyes. Crossed eyes.

DISQUALIFY: Yellow eyes. White locket or button. Visible tail kink.

TONKINESE COLORS

NATURAL MINK: **Body**—Medium brown. Ruddy highlight acceptable. **Points**—Dark brown. **Nose leather**—Dark brown (corresponding to the intensity of the point color). **Paw Pads**—Medium to dark brown (may have a rosy undertone).

CHAMPAGNE MINK: **Body**—Buff-cream. **Points**—Medium brown. **Nose leather**—Cinnamon-brown (corresponding to the intensity of the point color). **Paw pads**—Cinnamon-pink to cinnamon-brown.

BLUE MINK: **Body**—Soft, blue-gray with warm overtones. **Points**—Slate blue, distinctly darker than the body color. **Nose leather**—Blue-gray (corresponding to the intensity of the point color). **Paw pads**—Blue-gray (may have a rosy undertone).

PLATINUM MINK: **Body**—Pale, silvery gray with warm overtones. Not white or cream. **Points**—Frosty gray, distinctly darker than the body color. **Nose leather**—Lavender-pink to lavender-gray. **Paw pads**—Lavender-pink.

Tonkinese allowable outcross breeds: None.

TURKISH ANGORA

AUTHOR'S NOTE: The Turkish Angora is a fastidiously clean animal and prefers an immaculate home environment. Although this is a playful cat, and quite sociable with its family, it does better in a home where it is the star attraction and is not asked to share the spotlight with another cat. It is an intelligent and affectionate pet and likes what all cats like—close contact and good food served on time. The Turkish Angora hails from Ankara (Angora), Turkey. The true Angora was near extinction in the early twentieth century, as it was being replaced by Angoras crossed with Persians. It is one of the oldest longhair breeds and has been long admired in its homeland. The zoo in Ankara is credited for carefully preserving the white Angora for many decades of the twentieth century, until it was brought to North America in 1962, which helped to establish the breed as we know it today. It was accepted for registration by the CFA in 1970 and advanced to championship status in 1973.

The CFA only accepts for registration Turkish Angora imports that were born in the Ankara Zoo.

CFA Show Standards

POINT SCORE

HEAD	35
BODY	30
COLOR	20
COAT	15

GENERAL: Solid, firm, giving the impression of grace and flowing movement.

HEAD: Size, small to medium. Wedge-shaped. Wide at top. Definite taper toward chin. Allowance to be made for jowls in stud cat.

EARS: Wide at base, long, pointed, and tufted. Set high on the head and erect.

EYES: Large, almond-shaped. Slanting upward slightly.

NOSE: Medium-long, gentle slope. No break.

NECK: Slim and graceful, medium length.

CHIN: Gently rounded. Tip to form a perpendicular line with the nose.

JAW: Tapered.

BODY: Medium size in the female, slightly larger in the male. Torso long, graceful, and lithe. Chest, lightly framed. Rump slightly higher than front. Bone, fine.

LEGS: Long. Hind legs longer than front.

PAWS: Small and round, dainty. Tufts between toes.

TAIL: Long and tapering, wide at base, narrow at end, full. Carried lower than body but not trailing. When moving, relaxed tail is carried horizontally over the body, sometimes almost touching the head.

COAT: Body coat medium-long, long at ruff. Full brush on tail. Silky, with a wavy tendency. Wavier on stomach. Very fine and having a silklike sheen.

BALANCE: Proportionate in all physical aspects, with graceful, lithe appearance.

DISQUALIFY: Persian body type. Kinked or abnormal tail.

TURKISH ANGORA COLORS

White, black, blue, cream, red, black smoke, blue smoke, classic tabby pattern, mackerel tabby pattern, silver tabby, red tabby, brown tabby, blue tabby, cream tabby, tortoiseshell, calico, dilute calico, blue-cream, and bi-color.

OTAC (Other Turkish Angora Colors): Any other color or pattern with the exception of those showing hybridization resulting in the colors chocolate, lavender, the Himalayan pattern, or these combinations with white. **Eye color**—amber.

Turkish Angora allowable outcross breeds: None.

GLOSSARY

AGOUTI: Hairs that are banded with color, usually found between the stripes of a tabby coat pattern and other coat patterns.

AILUROPHILE: A lover of cats.

AILUROPHOBE: A detester of cats, or one who fears them.

ALTERED: Describes a cat that has been surgically sterilized.

ANGORA: Ancient name of the capital city of Turkey (Ankara). Archaic term for the first longhair cats seen in Europe. Recognized by most cat associations as Turkish Angora.

AOC: Any Other Color. Refers to colors other than those listed.

AOV: Any Other Variety. Refers to registered cats that are eligible to compete in show competition, but do not conform to the accepted show standard.

BARRING: Linear markings of the tabby (striped) coat pattern.

BAT-EARED: Having unusually large ears.

BI-COLORED: Having solid-color coat with patches of white.

BLAZE: Color marking from forehead to nose. Usually white or contrasting color of the coat.

BLUE: A coat color that is essentially gray but ranges from pale-blue gray to slate gray. Found on many breeds.

BREAK: Where the nose meets the forehead.

BRINDLING: Wrong-colored hairs intermingling with those of the correct color.

BRUSH: Profuse tail of a long-haired cat.

BUTTERFLY: Markings shaped like a butterfly found on the shoulders of well-marked tabby coat patterns.

BUTTON: A patch of color anywhere on the body, usually in white or contrasting color to the coat.

CALICO: A tortoiseshell with white color pattern. (See TORTOISESHELL.)

CAMEO: A white undercoat with red hair-tips.

CASTRATION: The surgical removal of the testes.

CAT FANCY: All those, as a group, involved in any aspect of breeding, showing, or promoting pure-breed cats.

CHAMPAGNE: A coat color that ranges from pale brownish gold to buff-cream.

CHAMPION: A title given to a cat having attained a designated number of wins at cat shows. (See PREMIER.)

CHINCHILLA: A coat with contrasting colors at the hair ends but lightly tipped.

CINNAMON: A light brown coat color resembling cinnamon.

CLASSIC TABBY: Refers to dense, clearly defined markings on the body that are darker than the ground color. They are unbroken on top and swirled on the sides, with rings on the tail and bars on the legs. The face is barred with upward-pointing lines, forming the letter M on the forehead.

COBBY: A heavy, low-lying, short-legged, compact, broad-chested, feline body type.

DILUTE: The paler hue or dilution of a color. Gray (or blue) is the dilution of black, etc.

DOUBLE COAT: Two layers of hair: a soft, thick undercoat and a slightly longer and thicker top coat.

EXOTIC: Breed type that is a cross between a Persian and various shorthair breeds.

FAWN: Coat color that ranges from rosy to pinkish beige.

FOREIGN: A long, tubular-shaped body type typified by the Siamese.

FRILL: The hair around the neck and down the chest that frames the face of longhair cats. Also referred to as the "ruff."

GLOVES: White markings on the base of the paws of the Birman.

GRAND CHAMPION: A title greater than Champion, awarded to a cat who has attained a designated number of wins in the Champion Class at cat shows. (See GRAND PREMIER.)

GRAND PREMIER: The equivalent of Grand Champion for a neutered or spayed cat.

GUARD HAIR: Long, stiff outer hair protecting the undercoat.

HAW: A third eyelid at the side or lower lid of the eye that slides horizontally from the inner corner. Seen when a cat is asleep or sick.

INBREEDING: Mating cats closely related to each other, such as brother to sister.

KINK: A malformed tail that is shortened and bent. Usually a birth defect.

LACES: The white markings (gloves) on the back paws that grow up from behind on the Birman.

LINE BREEDING: Mating of close members of the family, as mother and son, or grandfather and daughter, and so on, to produce a desired feature.

LOCKET: A patch of color under the neck that is white or in contrast to the base color of the coat.

MACKEREL TABBY: Refers to dense, clearly defined vertical stripes going around the body. The stripes are narrower than those of the Classic Tabby. The legs are striped with bracelets, and the tail is barred. The head is also barred, the bars forming the letter M on the forehead. The stripes often resemble those of a tiger.

MASK: Darker color hair on the face of pointed cats, such as the Siamese.

MUTATION: A genetic term indicating a radical physical change in a cat from birth, which can lead to the creation of a new breed. The twisted ears of the American Curl or the folded ears of the Scottish Fold are important examples.

MUZZLE: The cat's nose and jaws.

NEUTER: To surgically sterilize a cat.

NOSE LEATHER: The outer skin of the nose.

ODD-EYED: Having eyes of two different colors, usually blue and copper.

ORIENTAL: A descriptive term for breeds of a specific type, the most representative breed being the Siamese.

OUTCROSS: Mating unrelated cats of the same breed.

PADS: The soft tufts of skin under the paws.

PARTI-COLOR: A coat pattern with two separate colors.

PATCHED: Having random markings of different coloring on the coat.

PATCHED TABBY: Tabby patterns with random markings of red or cream.

PEKE-FACED: Resembling the face of a Pekingese dog. Short, depressed nose, indented between the eyes, with a wrinkled muzzle. Seen on Persian types.

PENCILLING: Pencil-like markings on the faces of cats with tabby coat patterns.

POINTS: The dark coloring on the cat's extremities, which include the head, legs, ears, and tail, as on a Siamese. Also, marks earned in cat shows according to breed standards.

POLYDACTYL: A cat with six or more toes on the front feet, five or more on the back feet.

PREMIER: A title won by neutered cats in cat shows that is the equivalent of Champion.

PURE-BREED: A cat produced from a line of cats of the same breed. Its lineage must be verified with a pedigree issued from a cat registering association.

QUEEN: A female cat that has become the mother of kittens.

RED: A vivid color that is more orange than actual red.

RINGS: Bands of color circling the legs or tail.

ROMAN NOSE: Nose with a high, prominent bridge. Seen in some Siamese and Rex.

RUDDY: A coat color associated with the Abyssinian that is orange-brown and ticked with dark brown or black.

RUFF: See FRILL.

SELF: A coat of solid color. Each hair is consistently the same color, from its tip to its root, and is the same on all parts of the body.

SHADED: Coat coloring in which the tips of the hairs are colored and the rest are white or pale. (See TIPPED.)

SHELL: A white undercoat with color at the tips of the hair shafts. Gives the appearance of a white or light-colored cat with a faint tinge of color.

SMOKE: White undercoat with colored hair-tips spreading down the hair shafts in an intense shade. White undercoat is not seen until the cat moves.

SNUB: Short nose type, such as that of the Persian.

SPAY: To surgically sterilize a female cat.

SPOTTED: A tabby coat pattern that is broken up, giving the appearance of spots rather than stripes.

SPRAY: A urinating habit of male cats, with implications of territorial marking and sexual announcements.

STOP: An abrupt change in the profile of the nose.

STUD BOOK: The official record of breeding for pure-breed cats, maintained by a registry organization. Stud books are now kept in computerized files.

TABBY: Coat patterns of specific types involving stripes, spots, or variations of stripes. Tabby types include Classic, Mackerel, Spotted, and Ticked.

TICKING: The bands of contrasting color on each hair shaft, as seen on Abyssinians.

TORBIE: A tortoiseshell with tabby patches.

TORTIE: See TORTOISESHELL.

TORTOISESHELL: A black coat color with patches of red (orange). It can also include dilute creams.

TUFTS: Slight clumps of hair growing from between the toes or on the ears.

UNDERCOAT: Shorter, softer hair lying under the top coat, found on double-coated cats.

VAN: Almost white coat, with patches of color on the head, tail, or legs. Also known as *Piebald*.

WEDGE: A head shape of various oriental breeds, such as the Siamese.

WHIP: A long, tapering tail.